Dear Reader,

Through our many years working as registered dietitians and certified diabetes care and education specialists, we have seen firsthand the toll that insulin resistance can take on health. If it is not addressed promptly and effectively, progression to pre-diabetes and ultimately type 2 diabetes is very possible. The good news is that taking action in the form of lifestyle changes can stop insulin resistance in its tracks. We have helped many clients **improve their health** and **reduce insulin resistance** by changing their dietary habits, increasing physical activity, and making other key lifestyle changes such as reducing stress, improving sleep, and getting needed resources and support. These changes work!

To reach a greater audience, we decided to write this book, sharing important information to help you better understand insulin resistance and how you can reverse it. We have worked hard to craft a **wide variety of recipes** for you not only to enjoy cooking and eating but also to help foster good health at the same time. Taking action is the first step toward halting the progression of insulin resistance. It is our sincere hope that the information in this book supports you on your path to managing your insulin resistance, while empowering you to develop lifelong healthy habits. We congratulate you for buying this book to help you take that first step on your journey.

Marie Feldman, RD, CDCES
Jodi Dalyai, MS, RD, CDCES

Welcome to the Everything® Series!

These handy, accessible books give you all you need to tackle a difficult project, gain a new hobby, comprehend a fascinating topic, prepare for an exam, or even brush up on something you learned back in school but have since forgotten.

You can choose to read an Everything® book from cover to cover or just pick out the information you want from our four useful boxes: Questions, Facts, Alerts, and Essentials. We give you everything you need to know on the subject, but throw in a lot of fun stuff along the way too.

question	fact
Answers to common questions.	Important snippets of information.

alert	essential
Urgent warnings.	Quick handy tips.

We now have more than 600 Everything® books in print, spanning such wide-ranging categories as cooking, health, parenting, personal finance, wedding planning, word puzzles, and so much more. When you're done reading them all, you can finally say you know Everything®!

PUBLISHER Karen Cooper

MANAGING EDITOR Lisa Laing

COPY CHIEF Casey Ebert

PRODUCTION EDITOR Jo-Anne Duhamel

ACQUISITIONS EDITOR Lisa Laing

DEVELOPMENT EDITOR Sarah Doughty

EVERYTHING® SERIES COVER DESIGNER Erin Alexander

THE
EVERYTHING®
GUIDE TO THE
INSULIN RESISTANCE DIET

**MARIE FELDMAN, RD, CDCES, AND
JODI DALYAI, MS, RD, CDCES**

LOSE WEIGHT, REVERSE INSULIN
RESISTANCE, AND STOP PRE-DIABETES

ADAMS MEDIA

NEW YORK   LONDON   TORONTO   SYDNEY   NEW DELHI

Aadamsmedia

Adams Media
An Imprint of Simon & Schuster, Inc.
100 Technology Center Drive
Stoughton, MA 02072

An Everything® Series Book.
Everything® and everything.com® are registered trademarks of Simon & Schuster, Inc.

First Adams Media trade paperback edition January 2021

ADAMS MEDIA and colophon are trademarks of Simon & Schuster.

For information about special discounts for bulk purchases, please contact Simon & Schuster Special Sales at 1-866-506-1949 or business@simonandschuster.com.

The Simon & Schuster Speakers Bureau can bring authors to your live event. For more information or to book an event contact the Simon & Schuster Speakers Bureau at 1-866-248-3049 or visit our website at www.simonspeakers.com.

Interior design by Colleen Cunningham
Photographs by James Stefiuk

Manufactured in China

10 9 8 7 6 5 4 3

Library of Congress Cataloging-in-Publication Data has been applied for.

ISBN 978-1-5072-1420-6
ISBN 978-1-5072-1421-3 (ebook)

Always follow safety and commonsense cooking protocols while using kitchen utensils, operating ovens and stoves, and handling uncooked food. If children are assisting in the preparation of any recipe, they should always be supervised by an adult.

The information in this book should not be used for diagnosing or treating any health problem. Not all diet and exercise plans suit everyone. You should always consult a trained medical professional before starting a diet, taking any form of medication, or embarking on any fitness or weight training program. The author and publisher disclaim any liability arising directly or indirectly from the use of this book.

Contains material adapted from the following titles published by Adams Media, an Imprint of Simon & Schuster, Inc.: *The Big Book of Diabetic Recipes* by Marie Feldman, RD, CDE, copyright © 2016, ISBN 978-1-4405-9365-9; *The Everything® DASH Diet Cookbook* by Christy Ellingsworth and Murdoc Khaleghi, MD, copyright © 2012, ISBN 978-1-4405-4353-1; *The Everything® Diabetes Cookbook, 2nd Edition* by Gretchen Scalpi, RD, CDN, CDE, copyright © 2010, ISBN 978-1-4405-0154-8; *The Everything® Guide to Managing and Reversing Pre-Diabetes, 2nd Edition* by Gretchen Scalpi, RD, CDN, CDE, copyright © 2013, ISBN 978-1-4405-5761-3; *The Everything® Guide to Managing Type 2 Diabetes* by Paula Ford-Martin with Jason Baker, MD, copyright © 2013, ISBN 978-1-4405-5196-3; *The Everything® Pre-Diabetes Cookbook* by Gretchen Scalpi, RD, CDN, CDE, copyright © 2014, ISBN 978-1-4405-7223-4; and *Healthy Habits for Managing & Reversing Prediabetes* by Marie Feldman, RD, copyright © 2019, ISBN 978-1-5072-0994-3.

Contents

Acknowledgments

A sincere thank you to Adams Media/Simon & Schuster for providing us with the opportunity to work on this project that centers on such an important topic. Thank you to our editor, Lisa Laing, who guided us throughout this venture, always providing timely feedback.

Professionally, I am very grateful to work under David Weingard, who is an inspirational leader to myself and all the wonderful staff and clients we work with at Cecelia Health, where we pride ourselves in making a difference in the lives of those with pre-diabetes and diabetes. Also, thank you to Dr. David Kayne, a wonderful mentor who has taught me so much about successfully diagnosing and treating pre-diabetes and diabetes through the patient care and clinical research we have conducted together over the years. Many thanks to my husband, Ken—you are my best friend, and I treasure our relationship, in which we motivate and elevate each other every day. I also want to express my heartfelt gratitude to my parents, who have given me ultimate unconditional love and support throughout my life in countless ways. I lovingly acknowledge my daughter Gabrielle, who inspires me every day to work hard to create a balanced, active, healthy, and happy life for our family. —MF

I am a published author due to my amazing friend and colleague, Marie. Thanks for inviting me to come along on this fun journey, sharing our life's work we both so deeply believe in. My nutrition and diabetes management experiences were developed and guided over the years by many amazing health educators, nurses, doctors, and myriad staff I was blessed to work with from Kaiser Permanente, UCLA, Cecelia Health, and Henry Mayo Newhall Hospital. Somehow, I had the good fortune to learn while young that nutrition and exercise were important to my health and those of others. Thank you to my parents, JoAlla and Don Gold, who showed me the power of education, curiosity, and hard work, and continue to support me on every adventure I choose to take. Thank you to my brother Seth Gold, whom I know is the better writer, whose vast intellect and uncle skills inspire me. My formal education into nutrition didn't start until adulthood, when I had the amazing support of my husband, Stephan. Thank you for letting me follow my dream and for living it with me, *én szeretlek*. My children Zoli and Erzsi act as my official taste testers, and always remind me that a healthy lifestyle isn't just healthy food. Your love, laughter, energy, and creativity are my true life force. —JD

Introduction

If you are reading this book, odds are that you or someone you know has concerns about insulin resistance. Insulin resistance means that the cells in your liver, muscles, and fat begin to have difficulty taking up glucose from the bloodstream because they don't respond well to, or resist, the insulin your body makes. In response, your pancreas makes more and more insulin to try to get the glucose into the weakened cells. Without changes to your diet and exercise level, your pancreas will eventually lose the battle, and the excess glucose will stay in your bloodstream. The increased blood sugar levels can lead to a diagnosis of pre-diabetes.

Many people know that they need to "do something" about their health, but are not sure where to begin or what to focus on, and until something goes wrong, there seems no need for urgency. Luckily, *The Everything® Guide to the Insulin Resistance Diet* provides a variety of tips, recipes, and a 10-week plan to help you manage—and even reverse— your insulin resistance. Even if you don't have insulin resistance and just want to keep up a healthy lifestyle to prevent it, this book will help. In Chapter 1, you'll explore the basics of insulin resistance, from its causes to its effects on the body. In Chapters 2 and 3, you'll discover how you can make changes that stop insulin resistance, as well as a simple plan for modifying your eating habits in busy everyday life. Chapters 4 and 5 offer more lifestyle changes you can make over time, including easy ways to work exercise into your schedule. And once you've taken a closer look into insulin resistance, check out the following chapters for 125 recipes to improve your health without sacrificing taste. From Bacon and Egg Breakfast Fried Rice and Spicy Almond Dip, to Sweet and Sour Pork Skillet and Double Chocolate Macaroons, these easy, mouthwatering recipes have every meal covered.

With new habits in place, and delicious, healthy recipes in your arsenal, you'll be on your way. You'll learn how to manage and possibly reverse insulin resistance, and you will also have adopted a healthier lifestyle, making you feel better in every way. If you're already doing things that are good for your health, you'll see how to maintain them and turn them into routines. Now let's get started with the information you need about insulin resistance and how healthy habits will help you reverse it.

CHAPTER 1

Insulin Resistance, Pre-Diabetes, and Diabetes

The best place to start when dealing with insulin resistance is to learn more about the condition, from how it affects your body to the risk factors that can offer clues as to how it may have become a reality for you (or why you may have a chance of developing it if you don't take action). When you understand insulin resistance and its part in your life, you understand the importance of seeking treatment with a medical professional, managing symptoms, and reducing risk through better lifestyle choices.

In this chapter, you will explore the physiology and science behind how insulin resistance develops and its impact on your body. You will discover more about its symptoms and what sets it apart from diabetes and pre-diabetes, as well as the different risk factors for developing insulin resistance. You will also find information about how to partner with your medical team to correctly diagnose and treat insulin resistance. Your journey to better health begins here.

Insulin Resistance and Its Impact on the Body

Insulin resistance is a condition where the body is unable to use its own insulin properly. Insulin, a hormone made by the pancreas, helps the body to use glucose, or blood sugar, for energy. People with insulin resistance require, and may produce, more insulin to help glucose get into cells. A consistent over-production of insulin, coupled with taking in more calories from food than you use, promotes weight gain. Eventually, the pancreas is no longer able to keep up with insulin demand, and blood glucose begins to rise to the pre-diabetic, or even diabetic, range.

alert

Insulin resistance may increase your risk of stroke. One study led by Dr. Tatjana Rundek and published in 2010 showed a strong relationship with insulin resistance and first-time ischemic stroke risk. In the study, those who tested in the top quarter of insulin resistance were at an increased risk for stroke, over any other vascular event. These results were stronger in men than women.

Genetic factors can play a part in insulin resistance. Perhaps you inherited a mutation in insulin receptors or glucose transporters, causing problems with the way your body manages and metabolizes blood glucose. Numerous genetic variations may interfere with how successful your body is at using insulin. And as you age, changes to your ability to produce glucose transporters can be a main cause of insulin resistance.

In other cases, people may require medications that can cause insulin resistance as a side effect. Research also continues to look at a variety of dietary factors as well, such as a possible connection between higher intake of sodium as a contributor to insulin resistance.

Ultimately, the most common cause of insulin resistance is obesity, meaning having too much fat stored in the body, and, in particular, having a higher than acceptable waist circumference.

Visceral fat, the fat stored in the abdomen, is more closely related to insulin resistance because this fat is stored in major organs, particularly the liver. The liver is responsible for complicated aspects of your metabolic system, and when glucose isn't properly utilized, it cannot perform these functions. Visceral fat increases inflammation and leads to a disruption of the entire body's insulin signaling. Muscle, organ, and fat cells all take in varying amounts of glucose for energy via insulin. The ability of these cells to make energy, and ultimately do their individual jobs, is therefore affected when insulin fails to get glucose into the cell. When someone gains weight, the excess fat is stored not only in fat tissue but also in cells throughout the body, including organs and muscles. The accumulation of fat in these cells impairs the insulin signaling. Impairing insulin's ability to work on cells leads to the overproduction of insulin, excess glucose in the bloodstream, the eventual storage of this energy as fat, and, ultimately, increased inflammation and eventual disease.

The Pancreas: A Key Player in Insulin Production

Insulin resistance has to do with the endocrine system, so understanding how the pancreas functions as part of this system helps to illustrate the way insulin resistance, pre-diabetes, and diabetes can develop.

The endocrine system is composed of glands that secrete hormones. Hormones travel through the circulatory system to regulate metabolism, growth, sexual development, and reproduction. If any of these glands secrete either too little or too much of a hormone, the entire body can be thrown off balance.

The pancreas is located in the abdomen, next to the upper part of the small intestine. It's long and tapered with a thicker bottom end (or head), which is cradled in the downward curve of the duodenum—a part of the small intestine. The long end (or tail) of the pancreas extends up behind the stomach toward the spleen. A main duct connects the pancreas to the duodenum.

A Tale of Two Pancreatic Functions

The pancreas performs two major functions in the body, which are carried out by two different types of cells located within the organ. These cells allow it to pull double duty as both a digestive organ and a regulator of energy balance and metabolism. Sitting behind the stomach, the pancreas secretes both digestive enzymes and endocrine hormones.

The exocrine portion of the pancreas is primarily involved with digestion. Exocrine cells in the pancreas secrete digestive enzymes into the duodenum. There the enzymes help process carbohydrates, proteins, and other nutrients. The other group of cells is the pancreatic endocrine tissue.

The endocrine pancreas accounts for a very small part of the organ, but it contains key cell clusters—islets of Langerhans—constructed of various cell types that each make and secrete a different hormone.

> **fact**
>
> Islets (pronounced EYE-lets) of Langerhans are named after Dr. Paul Langerhans, a German physician who first described them in medical literature in 1869. A normal human pancreas can contain as many as one million islets, yet they amount to just about 1–2 percent of the total mass of the pancreas.

The three main types of cells in the endocrine pancreas are:

1. **Alpha cells.** These manufacture and release glucagon, a hormone that raises blood glucose levels.

2. **Beta cells.** These monitor blood sugar levels and produce insulin-lowering glucose in response.
3. **Delta cells.** These produce the hormone somatostatin, which researchers believe is responsible for directing the action of both the beta and alpha cells.

The endocrine part of the pancreas is the one to watch as far as pre-diabetes and diabetes are concerned.

The Liver-Pancreas Partnership

The liver, located toward the front of the abdomen and above the stomach, is critical to the insulin resistance story. The liver is the center of glucose storage. It converts glucose—the fuel that the cells of the human body require for energy—into its principal storage form, glycogen. Glycogen is stored in muscles and in the liver itself, where it can later be converted back to glucose for energy with the help of the hormones epinephrine (secreted by the adrenal glands) and glucagon (from the alpha cells of the pancreas). Together, the liver and pancreas preserve a delicate balance of blood glucose and insulin, produced in sufficient amounts to both fuel cells and maintain glycogen storage.

Insulin and Blood Sugar

While the liver is one source of glucose, most of the glucose the body uses is manufactured from food, primarily carbohydrates. Cells then convert blood glucose from food into energy. Insulin is the hormone that makes it all happen. When you eat a meal containing carbohydrates, they are broken down to glucose in the blood. Often referred to as *carbs*, carbohydrates include starchy foods such as bread, rice, cereal, pasta, and sweets, as well as fruit and some vegetables. The increase in your blood glucose, a.k.a. *blood sugar*, signals the pancreas to release insulin, and this hormone allows the sugar to move from the blood into cell tissues, such as the muscles, fat cells, and the liver, where it can be used for energy or stored as glycogen or fat.

Causes and Risk Factors for Insulin Resistance

There are a variety of reasons why someone may develop insulin resistance. Understanding these factors in more detail can help you understand why you may have been diagnosed with the condition or are at risk of potentially developing it. The main causes and risk factors for insulin resistance include:

- Excess weight
- Age (45 years of age or older)
- Family history of insulin resistance, pre-diabetes, or diabetes
- Physical inactivity
- Smoking
- High blood pressure and elevated cholesterol levels
- History of gestational diabetes
- Polycystic ovary syndrome (PCOS)
- Other risk factors (medications, disorders, sleep problems)

Let's take a look at these risk factors in more detail.

Excess Weight

Too much fat makes it difficult for the body to use its own insulin to process blood glucose and bring it down to normal circulating levels. The specifics are as follows:

Overweight people have fewer available insulin receptors, and the effectiveness of the receptors is hampered by the storage of excess free fatty acids (FFAs), broken down during fat metabolism and released in the circulation, in muscle and organ cells rather than fat cells. When compared to muscle cells, fat cells have fewer insulin receptors where the insulin binds with the cell and "unlocks" it to process glucose into energy. More fat requires more insulin. The pancreas starts producing larger and larger quantities of insulin in order to "feed" body mass and override the ineffective insulin receptors, and consequently insulin resistance turns into a vicious circle.

> **fact**
>
> Obesity and body fat in adults are measured by body mass index (BMI)—a number that expresses weight in relationship to your height and is a reliable indicator of overall body fat. People with a BMI of 25–29.9 are considered overweight; those with a BMI of 30 or over are obese. You should aim for a BMI of 18.5–24.9, which is considered normal.

Excess blood sugar must be stored as fat, and excess fat promotes further insulin resistance. Fat cells release FFAs during lipolysis (the breakdown of fat within cells). FFAs are released into the bloodstream, interfering with glucose metabolism. Abdominal fat appears to release higher levels of FFAs than other parts of the body, leading to the dangers associated with higher visceral or "belly" fat storage. Luckily, visceral fat decreases early on in initial weight loss.

Age

With age, muscle mass declines and fat mass increases. Excess fat leads to insulin resistance. Changes within the body over time may also contribute to insulin resistance. For example, the liver may become less sensitive to signaling to store rather than release glucose, leading to the overproduction of insulin. The production of one of the major glucose transport proteins, GLUT4, also declines with age. With decreased GLUT4, insulin receptors on cell membranes are less effective, continuing the cycle of pancreatic burnout. Other age-related changes to the body, such as increased inflammation, may contribute. Maintaining muscle mass becomes paramount as a cornerstone of reducing risk for insulin resistance.

Family History

There is strong evidence that multiple genetic factors could put a person at risk for insulin resistance and the resulting risks of pre-diabetes and diabetes. Genetic variants have been discovered that alter the effectiveness of hormone receptors, beta cell function, and insulin secretion.

Obesity has the strongest influence on insulin resistance. It is possible that as many as 43 percent of people have a gene referred to as *FTO* for fat mass and obesity. This gene may make it harder for a person to control overeating, and they may continue to feel hungry despite an adequate diet. It may also lead to a predisposition to store more fat or be less active. Developing strategies to combat sedentary behaviors, hunger cues, and food choices are critical to overcoming a family history of obesity, insulin resistance, and diabetes.

Physical Inactivity

A sedentary lifestyle is one of the biggest contributors to insulin resistance. Research shows that after just one bout of exercise, the utilization of glucose increases throughout the body and this effect can last as long as 48 hours. Interestingly, the impact that exercise has on blood sugar improvement dwindles in both average people and athletes within the same time frame. If someone who exercises regularly stops, within 2–3 days they have a 50 percent reduction in insulin sensitivity; thus lack of physical activity contributes to insulin resistance. Physical activity is also a major component of weight control, and lack of activity contributes to obesity.

Smoking

While smoking rates in the US have continued to go down over the years, as much as 15 percent of the population still smokes. While many are aware of the risks it poses to heart health and cancer, insulin resistance and diabetes may not be the most obvious result of smoking. Studies of weight and fat storage in smokers versus nonsmokers show that while smokers tend to have lower weights, except for heavy smokers, changes take place that lead to storage of fat in the abdomen. Hormone changes that take place in both male and female smokers appear to cause the shift to increased abdominal fat storage, and this storage directly increases risk for insulin resistance.

High Blood Pressure and Elevated Cholesterol Levels

Hypertension, or high blood pressure, leads to extreme pressure being placed on the arteries. The delicate tissue lining the arteries, made of endothelial cells, becomes rigid and inflexible. Blood does not flow as freely and inflammation is increased, causing systemic problems throughout the body. Insulin resistance is one result of the impairment of blood movement with hypertension.

When cholesterol is elevated, excess lipids are traveling in the blood, further reducing the effectiveness of your vascular system—the network of arteries and veins that carries oxygen, along with glucose and other nutrients, around the body. Increased cholesterol synthesis in the liver (meaning the liver makes a higher amount of cholesterol in the body) is seen in those with insulin resistance, but mostly in those of a higher body mass index. High triglycerides (a type of fat) and low high-density lipoprotein (HDL) cholesterol (the "good" cholesterol) are regularly seen in those with insulin resistance. This combination is especially dangerous to the cardiovascular system and is strongly correlated with the development of type 2 diabetes.

History of Gestational Diabetes

Research suggests that women with a history of gestational diabetes, a form of diabetes that affects pregnant women, could be at up to 4.4 times the risk for developing insulin resistance within 2 years of their pregnancy. If a woman is obese prior to getting pregnant, and has gestational diabetes during the pregnancy, that risk increases by twenty-six times.

Polycystic Ovary Syndrome

Polycystic ovary syndrome (PCOS) affects approximately 5–10 percent of women in the US. PCOS is a grouping of reproductive health problems characterized by polycystic ("having many cysts") ovaries. It is the most common cause of irregular menstrual cycles and infertility. Most women with PCOS have insulin resistance and hyperinsulinism. Hyperinsulinism means that high amounts of insulin are routinely produced to combat the insulin resistance. Like metabolic syndrome, an overproduction of insulin triggers a cycle of easy weight gain.

Other Risk Factors

Taking certain medications such as glucocorticoids, antipsychotics, and some medicines for HIV can cause insulin resistance. Many different disorders, such as Werner syndrome, Cushing's syndrome, and acromegaly, and hormone therapies such as androgen deprivation therapy used in prostate cancer treatment can also cause insulin resistance.

Sleep problems also put you at risk. Lack of sleep triggers a rise in cortisol (the stress hormone) and other hormones, making the body less sensitive to insulin. In obstructive sleep apnea, or OSA, a combination of loss of sleep along with a deprivation in oxygen during sleep can lead to insulin resistance.

Signs and Symptoms of Insulin Resistance

Unfortunately, some people with insulin resistance may have no signs or symptoms at all, but for others, possible signs or symptoms to look out for are:

1. **Feeling Tired.** Overall low energy can be a result of insulin resistance. If you are not able to get glucose into your cells to make energy, you may not have enough for your day-to-day needs.
2. **Visceral Fat.** Having an apple-shaped body, with excess pounds packed in the midsection rather than the hips, is another hallmark of insulin resistance. In fact, the National Institutes of Health recommends that waist circumference be

used as a screening tool for evaluating the risk of heart disease and type 2 diabetes.

3. **Excess Hunger.** It can be hard to determine which comes first, but when the body is deprived of energy due to insulin not getting the glucose into cells, the results can also be that you have increased hunger as your body seeks the energy it needs.

4. **Acanthosis Nigricans.** Excess insulin in the blood can cause skin cells to overproduce, creating thick, darkened patches of skin in certain areas of the body, such as the back of the neck, underarms, or groin area. Other conditions may cause this skin condition, so if you notice these skin changes, it is important to see a physician.

5. **Other Signs of Metabolic Syndrome.** If you have elevated triglycerides, elevated cholesterol, hypertension, low HDL cholesterol, and/or elevated blood sugars, you may also have insulin resistance.

Again it is important to keep in mind that you may or may not show symptoms of insulin resistance. If you have one or more of these symptoms, you may want to consult your doctor about getting tested. And if you do not have any symptoms but have risk factors, it is always a good idea to discuss monitoring for its development with your medical team.

Pre-Diabetes and Diabetes

To visualize the role of insulin in the body and in pre-diabetes and diabetes, think of a flattened basketball. The ball needs air (in the body's case, glucose) to supply the necessary energy to bounce. To fill a basketball, you insert an inflating needle into the ball valve to open it, then pump air into the ball. Likewise, when a cell needs energy, insulin binds to an insulin receptor, or cell gateway, to "open" the cell and let glucose in for processing. You can blow pounds and pounds of compressed air at the ball valve, but without a needle to open it, the air will not enter. The same applies to your cells. Without insulin to bind to the receptors and open the cell for glucose, the glucose cannot enter. Instead, it builds up to damaging levels in the bloodstream.

In people with insulin resistance, that progresses to pre-diabetes and eventually type 2 diabetes, as the pancreatic beta cells start to "burn out" and die, resulting in insulin insufficiency (also known as *insulin deficiency*). Researchers have hypothesized that those who have progressed to type 2 diabetes at diagnosis may have lost as much as 90 percent of their beta cell function.

What Makes Pre-Diabetes Different from Type 2 Diabetes?

The term *pre-diabetes* was introduced by the American Diabetes Association (ADA) in 2002 as a way to more clearly describe a state that is between normal blood sugar and type 2 diabetes. In the past, your doctor may have diagnosed you with "borderline diabetes." Before 2002, your doctor might have told you, "your blood sugar is a little high," or "you have a touch of sugar." These words provide little meaning to the person hearing them, and they don't show the urgent need to do something about the situation. Pre-diabetes is defined by specific boundaries, namely the results of blood glucose tests.

When you have pre-diabetes, your blood sugar level is higher than normal, but it's not yet high enough to be classified as type 2 diabetes. Pre-diabetes means that you are on your way to developing diabetes if there are no interventions on your part. *However,* progressing to type 2 diabetes is not inevitable. There is a great deal that you can do to reverse pre-diabetes and bring your blood sugar level back to a normal range. A diagnosis of type 2 diabetes, on the other hand, is permanent. While there is much that can be done to control diabetes, it is important to realize that type 2 diabetes does not go away.

If you have received a diagnosis of pre-diabetes, there is some good news. You have received a wake-up call and been given an opportunity to improve your health, lose weight, and make healthy lifestyle changes. If you take action now, you can prevent, or at the very least halt, the progression to a serious, more permanent disease.

Diagnosing Pre-Diabetes and Diabetes

If you are trying to determine whether you have pre-diabetes or diabetes or are monitoring your condition after you have been diagnosed, you will need to have some information about your health. This information includes lab tests, blood pressure, and other measurements such as weight and waist circumference. Three types of blood tests are used to diagnose pre-diabetes and diabetes: a fasting blood glucose test, an oral glucose tolerance test, and a hemoglobin A1c test. Your prior health history provides additional clues in the determination of pre-diabetes or diabetes.

FASTING BLOOD GLUCOSE TEST

A fasting blood glucose test provides a clue about the possibility of pre-diabetes. In this simple blood test taken at your doctor's office or lab, you have a sample of blood drawn first thing in the morning after an overnight fast.

> **alert**
>
> A fasting blood glucose test means just that: *fasting*. If you are having your blood test in the morning, you should not have anything to eat or drink (besides water) after midnight the night before. Refrain from doing exercise before your test, as that could also affect your reading, providing an inaccurate result.

A fasting blood glucose of 100mg/dl–125mg/dl on more than one occasion is an indicator for pre-diabetes, whereas a fasting blood glucose of 126mg/dl or above indicates diabetes.

TWO-HOUR ORAL GLUCOSE TOLERANCE TEST

Some doctors prefer using a glucose challenge rather than a fasting test. In this case, you are given a glucose drink that provides 75 grams of glucose. Blood is drawn 2 hours after taking the drink, and then the blood glucose is measured. With this test, a blood glucose result of 140mg/dl–199mg/dl 2 hours after taking 75 grams of glucose (on more than one occasion) indicates pre-diabetes.

Two-hour readings that are above 200mg/dl on more than one occasion indicate diabetes.

HEMOGLOBIN A1C TEST

When a fasting blood glucose test or 2-hour glucose challenge is done, the reading provides a result for that moment in time. Because your glucose can vary a great deal throughout the day, these tests do not provide information about what your blood sugar is at other times of the day or longer term. That is why a test called the *hemoglobin A1c (HbA1c)* is done, particularly when your doctor suspects pre-diabetes or diabetes.

Hemoglobin is a substance found in red blood cells that carries oxygen from the lungs to all cells in the body. When hemoglobin binds with glucose, glycated hemoglobin (or glycohemoglobin) is formed. The A1c portion of glycated hemoglobin is the easiest and largest portion of this compound to measure. A person with higher blood glucose has more glycated hemoglobin than someone with normal blood glucose. Hemoglobin found in red blood cells lasts for 60–90 days. As a result, when hemoglobin A1c is measured, the doctor can form a fairly accurate reflection of your average blood glucose levels over the last 60–90 days. A hemoglobin A1c between 5.7 and 6.4 percent indicates pre-diabetes, and a hemoglobin A1c of 6.5 percent and above indicates diabetes.

In addition to checking hemoglobin A1c blood sugar levels and fasting blood glucose levels at diagnosis, your doctor will likely check them at regular intervals thereafter to keep tabs on your progress. Monitoring your hemoglobin A1c and keeping it below 5.7 percent, and keeping fasting blood glucose levels close to 100mg/dl (or more specific targets determined for you individually by your medical team), should be part of your action plan.

Why Does Blood Sugar Need to Be Controlled?

Keeping your blood sugar levels under control is key to managing pre-diabetes and preventing adverse outcomes, such as the development of type 2 diabetes and all the potential complications that can go with it. A diagnosis of pre-diabetes does not mean you will automatically develop type 2 diabetes. If you take action early to get the right treatment to return blood sugars to normal range, you can avoid diabetes. However, the longer you let your blood sugars stay elevated, the greater your risk of progressing to type 2 diabetes.

The pancreas of a person who is on the fringe of type 2 diabetes generates insulin, but the body is unable to process it in sufficient amounts to control blood sugar levels. This inability is due to a problem with how the body's cells—specifically the insulin receptors that attract and process the hormone—recognize and use insulin. As blood sugar levels rise, the pancreas pumps out more and more insulin to try to compensate. This pumped insulin may bring blood sugar levels down to a degree, but it also results in high levels of circulating insulin, a condition known as *hyperinsulinemia*. At a certain threshold, the weakened pancreas cannot produce enough insulin, and over time beta cell mass is lost. As beta cells die, insulin deficiency develops. At this point, you move into type 2 diabetes. If you don't carefully control your blood sugars at this point, then both short- and long-term complications can develop.

The First Line of Defense: A Healthy Lifestyle

Multiple studies have shown that the best way to prevent/treat insulin resistance, as well as halt the progression of pre-diabetes and diabetes in those at risk, is through making and maintaining changes in lifestyle. Important lifestyle modifications such as weight loss (for those who are overweight or obese), a healthy diet, regular physical activity, adequate sleep, and stress management are considered the best and first-line approach.

CHAPTER 2

First Steps: Learn to Change Habits, Set Goals, and Lose Weight

Behavior has a powerful influence on health, so much so that even the most detailed and comprehensive lifestyle plan is destined to fail unless it includes a sound behavior modification component. A large part of behavioral change centers on your habits. Developing and focusing on the right kind of habits empowers you to turn your best intentions and the knowledge you have acquired about ways to change your lifestyle (such as diet and exercise) into a reality.

Learning more about habits, understanding the science behind them, and uncovering ways to develop healthy positive habits are all key to any lasting lifestyle changes, including managing insulin resistance. In this chapter, you will explore how habits form and how you can create good habits that will allow you to combat insulin resistance successfully.

What Is a Habit?

Habits are a major part of your everyday routine. From the time you get up in the morning until the time your head hits the pillow at night, your day is filled with countless actions and choices—almost half of which may be habits. In fact, the life of humans (and other living creatures) has been characterized largely as a "bundle of habits" by William James, a famous Harvard psychologist and philosopher who led some of the earliest investigations about the psychology and neurology behind habits in the late 1800s. Since then, numerous studies have been conducted into how habits are formed and maintained.

While the precise definition of *habit* has been debated, the most common definition revolves around the following concept: Habits are automatic behavioral responses to environmental cues or triggers.

How Do Habits Form?

There are countless theories as to how habits are learned and created, how they develop, and why they persist. One of the most common explanations of habit formation is offered by Ann Graybiel, PhD, an MIT professor who has conducted extensive research in the area of habits. Her explanation involves the following sequence of events:

1. First, you acquire a habit by experience(s) that leads to creation and organization of neuron connections in your brain.

2. Second, you repeat the habit behavior over time; do it enough, and it can become fixed.
3. Third, the habit is fully acquired, and you now perform it automatically, without requiring direct attention or focus.
4. Fourth, the habit becomes a sequence of actions that tends to occur in response to a particular situation or cue.

Essentially, once habits are learned, repeated, and acquired, they occur automatically. Things like preparing a cup of coffee or brushing your teeth, which you learned through a series of steps that required significant concentration and time, have been well integrated into your routine. Now you perform them with barely any thought.

> **question**
>
> **What is a cue?**
>
> A cue is an impulse or trigger that leads to a routine, such as a habit. Cues can be external (coming from your environment), or internal (coming from within). Examples of external cues are locations, times of day, or other people; for instance, going to the movies is a cue for the habit of eating popcorn. Internal cues include mood, thought patterns, and sensations in the body, such as the feeling of hunger making you want to eat.

We rely on habits because they allow us to perform a variety of actions in daily life, often while doing other things, without having to stop and fully concentrate on what we are doing—saving time and energy.

The Importance of Habits for Good Health

It's no secret that habits are key to health. They can make or break your chances of achieving and maintaining wellness goals such as eating right, staying fit, and managing insulin resistance and other medical conditions, along with increasing your quality of life and promoting longevity. Taking a look at your current habits, deciding what needs to be changed, and then learning how to increase positive habits, as well as reduce negative ones, is an important step toward helping you manage your insulin resistance and overall health.

Harnessing the Power of Habits

Making the decision to change your habits, namely decreasing the ones that are harmful and increasing or adding those that are beneficial, is a great first step toward managing your insulin resistance. But then how do you move forward to take action and change these habits? There are a number of strategies that can help you change and/or adopt habits for lifestyle change. Think about which of the following tips and techniques may be right for you, and remember: Trial and error, an open mind, and some patience will be key.

LEARN ALL YOU CAN TO PROMOTE CHANGE

You may be curious and want to modify your lifestyle, but you're not sure how. Studies have shown that education can help increase your intention and motivation to change, thus inspiring you to take action. Reading this book is a great start; the following chapters are chock-full of useful ideas and suggestions about ways to add more healthy habits to your routine. In addition, reaching out to a health professional, such as a registered dietitian and/or behavioral therapist to get one-on-one instruction can be another wonderful way to learn more.

PAY ATTENTION TO YOUR CUES AND ACTIONS

As you've discovered, a cue is an impulse or trigger that leads to a routine, such as a habit. Charles Duhigg, in his bestseller *The Power of Habit*, suggests that there is an actual "habit loop" you go through when developing and experiencing habits. It all starts with a cue. He describes a three-step process in the brain:

1. **Cue.** First there is a cue, an initiator that signals the brain to begin the habit.
2. **Routine.** Then comes a behavioral action that is taken as a result of the cue.
3. **Reward.** Finally, there is a benefit that is experienced as a result of the routine, which will reinforce the brain to encode the habit for continued use.

Identifying the cues that trigger your habits is an important beginning step to changing the behavior, namely bad habits.

Is there a certain time of day or place (like the couch!) when/where you tend to snack?

Does being with certain people cause you to stay out too late and miss sleep?

Do certain moods affect your ability to stick to your exercise routine?

Taking note of these cues can help you become aware of what leads you to engage in certain behaviors, so you can identify what you may be doing wrong as a result and ways you might change that. On the flip side, adding in certain cues to encourage new and positive health habit formation is important too, such as putting a large water bottle on your desk to prompt you to drink more or putting your gym clothes in the car to remind you to go to the gym after work.

In some cases, you may be able to change some of the cues, like avoiding certain environments or people that are bad influences, but changing the behavior that results from the cue and/or the reward is believed to be more realistic and beneficial.

In addition to the "habit loop," Duhigg also suggests a way to transform habits by using the "golden rule of habit change." This involves allowing the cue and the reward to remain the same and just changing the routine that connects them. For example, if you normally go out with your friends (cue) to eat somewhere that is not healthy (routine) mainly to enjoy their companionship (reward), instead you could spend time with friends in an activity not centered on food, like going for a walk or attending a concert, so you are able to enjoy the reward of their companionship without sabotaging your eating plan.

essential

A great deal of research has shown that keeping food and activity diaries can help promote healthy behavior—and noting specific cues that come before the behavior can be especially useful. A 2014 study conducted by A.A.C. Verhoeven and others showed that when participants kept a cue-monitoring diary, it helped decrease unhealthy snacking in comparison to those subjects using the control diary that did not focus on recording cues.

Developing a competing routine that is more positive and healthful can help bring about change that is good for you in response to your usual cues. And it will still yield a similar, if not the same, reward.

RETHINK YOUR REWARDS

Another strategy that has been proven to be successful with adopting healthy habits is to change the way you reward yourself, particularly if what you normally do is working against your attempts to change your lifestyle. If you commonly celebrate successes in life by using food as a reward, then keep the habit of celebrating an accomplishment, but replace the reward with a nonfood treat, such as a new book or a shopping trip with a friend. If you use TV time on the couch to indulge yourself after a long day, instead take a walk with a friend or enroll in a yoga class to relax and recharge.

REPEAT, REPEAT, REPEAT...

Research has shown time and time again that the more you repeat a behavioral routine, the more likely it is to become a habit. Use this concept to your advantage. If you know how to eat healthy, exercise, and make other lifestyle changes to manage your insulin resistance, then get out there and try it. Do it often—and then some! The more times you allow yourself to put your intentions and knowledge into practice via action, the easier it becomes. Repeating healthy behaviors increases skill, motivation, and confidence, which are all key to maintaining long-lasting habits for success.

LET YOUR HABITS BUILD ON EACH OTHER

If you tie a new healthy habit to an existing one, the potential for change and success multiplies. Some examples are:

- Going to bed early so it will be easier for you to wake up for your regular exercise class
- Grabbing a piece of fruit after your workout
- Drinking a big glass of water before your healthy meal

- Talking about your stressors with a friend while walking instead of sitting at the local coffee shop

Find opportunities to multitask in a good way to let your healthy habits build upon each other. This will increase motivation and expand your network of healthy habits.

SET YOURSELF UP FOR SUCCESS

Studies show that you are more likely to be successful with changing your behavior and sticking with a healthy habit if you not only are ready to change but also believe in yourself and have support. As you continue to learn and practice your habits, things will get easier and you will be able to take on new challenges and build on past successes—boosting your confidence along the way. You will also want to surround yourself with people who will elevate you to help you reach your goals, and minimize interactions with those who do not have your best interests in mind and only want to encourage old routines or bad habits.

Positive communication is of the utmost importance. If you are having trouble getting started, are lacking confidence in your abilities, or require more education to achieve your goals, reach out to your medical team, family, and friends to get the help and support you need to start. It will make a big difference in the beginning and throughout your journey to better health.

PLAN FOR CHALLENGES AND SETBACKS

When trying to change your habits and add new positive ones, remember that this is a process and that challenges and setbacks can happen. Some challenges you can plan for in advance, and others may present themselves out of the blue, and you will have to do your best to work to overcome them. Always keep in mind the value of keeping a positive attitude. Stress and negative thoughts are draining and have the potential to derail your efforts. They can make it difficult to maintain your healthy habits and can even lead to new bad habits or allow you to relapse to previous undesirable ones, so it is important for you to get a handle on them. Beware of the "all-or-nothing" attitude that can set you up for failure. If you make a mistake, realize that you are human, give yourself some credit, and try to learn from it. If you need help with working on stress management and coping techniques, as well as goal setting, working with a healthcare professional may be a good idea.

Goal Setting and a Healthy Lifestyle

When you are managing any chronic health condition, especially one that touches so many facets of your lifestyle, like having insulin resistance, it's important to have goals to work toward. Goals not only help you measure progress; they can also be incredibly empowering and motivational when they are set and tracked correctly. However, the wrong kind of goal setting can have the opposite effect. Goals that are unrealistic or too vague, or that don't hold you to any timeline for completion, may work against you. It may sound counterintuitive, but it may be helpful to initially set your sights low. If you aim for the stars relative to your starting point, you may become easily discouraged if you don't hit that big goal as quickly as you feel you should.

SMART Goals

In the long run, the most effective goals are SMART goals: specific, measurable, action-oriented, realistic, and timely.

1. **Specific.** Don't be vague or general. Saying "I will eat healthier" leaves a lot of room for interpretation. But saying "I will add one more serving of a low-carb vegetable to my meals each day for a week" is a concrete objective you can achieve.
2. **Measurable.** Make sure your goals can be measured against something. Whether it's testing blood sugar three more times a week or exercising 20 additional minutes a day, putting a number against your goal helps ensure you're making progress.
3. **Action-Oriented.** It may go without saying, but your goal should require you to do something to achieve it. Goals aren't wishes; they are something to work toward by taking tangible steps.
4. **Realistic.** Do not set goals you are simply not capable of making or goals that require too much drastic change at once. A realistic goal is something you are certain you can achieve in the short term.

5. **Timely.** Set a time limit for your goal. Starting with a short period can be a good motivator for sticking to your goal. As you experience success meeting it, you can always extend the time frame longer.

Start by picking one goal for yourself. If you're having problems figuring out what the best goal is for you to start with, you can work with your doctor, dietitian, or diabetes educator to narrow down the options.

When You Meet Your Goals

What's the best thing to do once you've met a SMART goal? Get SMARTER, of course! That means evaluating (E) and resetting (R) your goals. Look at the progress you've made with the original goal. How well did you do in achieving it? Are you satisfied with the results? Are there any changes you could make to do better the next time around in terms of being specific, measurable, action-oriented, realistic, and timely?

If you feel the goal you've worked toward and met has become a healthy new lifestyle habit, then it's time to move on to a new goal (with SMART goal setting in mind, of course). But if your achieved goal isn't quite habit yet, or if the time frame for your goal has elapsed without quite meeting the measurement you set for yourself, you might consider resetting to the same goal—with any modifications you figured out while evaluating your success (e.g., set a different time frame, determine a change in measure).

Remember that you can evaluate and reset goals at any time if you feel like you aren't making adequate progress. Goals should always be a work in progress. And you should always be working toward a goal, even if you've reached your target weight, blood sugars, or other desired health parameters. Doing so will help you stay motivated toward maintaining good health and prevent you from becoming complacent.

Weight Management

After all this talk of changing habits and setting goals, you may wonder where to start. One of the most important things you can do to combat insulin resistance is to reach or maintain a healthy weight. There is a significant link between excess weight and insulin resistance/blood sugar control. The best way to assess your weight status is determining your BMI. There are many BMI calculators online, or you can also do this with your healthcare provider. As shown in the following chart, adults with a BMI of 25–29.9 are considered overweight; those with a BMI of 30 or over are obese. Talk with your healthcare provider about your optimal BMI and goal weight. A general rule is to aim for a BMI under 25.

The most recent data from 2017 shows that 4 out of 10 adults in the US are obese, and the rate of childhood obesity is also skyrocketing with more than 18 percent of the nation's children classified as obese. Eighty percent of people with type 2 diabetes

BODY MASS INDEX (BMI)

Classification of Overweight and Obesity by BMI, Waist Circumference, and Associated Risk of Type 2 Diabetes, Hypertension, and Cardiovascular Disease

Classification	BMI	Disease Risk Relative to a Waist Circumference of ≤102 cm. (for men); ≤88 cm. (for women)	Disease Risk Relative to a Waist Circumference of >102 cm. (for men); >88 cm. (for women)
Underweight	<18.5	no increased risk	no increased risk
Normal	18.5–24.9	no increased risk	no increased risk
Overweight	25.0–29.9	increased	high
Obesity	30.0–34.9	high	very high
Obesity	35.0–39.9	very high	very high

are also overweight or obese. Luckily, there is strong evidence that managing obesity can improve insulin resistance and delay the progression of insulin resistance to pre-diabetes and diabetes. While losing weight is paramount to preventing or reversing insulin resistance, knowing where to start can be challenging.

The Benefits of Weight Loss

When beginning your weight loss journey, it can be both helpful and motivating to learn about all the health benefits of shedding excess pounds. Losing weight makes a big difference in your body's ability to control blood sugar. The Diabetes Prevention Program that started in 1996 proved that even modest weight loss, 5–10 percent of body weight, can prevent or delay the onset of type 2 diabetes in overweight at-risk adults.

Precisely how excess fat promotes insulin resistance isn't entirely clear, but it is thought that fat stored within muscle and organ cells, intracellular fat, impairs the triggering of insulin receptors. If receptors on cell membranes do not appropriately connect with insulin or if they impede the insulin from opening the cell membrane, then glucose doesn't get out of the blood and into the cells to make energy. In addition, research has found that the "apple-shaped" body (central abdominal obesity) associated with insulin resistance and type 2 diabetes contains fat with unique properties. Specifically, this type of visceral abdominal fat sheds more free fatty acids, which can elevate triglyceride levels, and is associated with higher insulin levels that promote further fat storage. Paring down abdominal fat will have the double benefit of both increasing insulin sensitivity and decreasing triglyceride levels in people with insulin resistance, pre-diabetes, and type 2 diabetes. If you are overweight, keep in mind that even modest weight loss can decrease insulin resistance and improve control.

In addition to keeping your insulin resistance in check, there are numerous other health benefits to losing weight, including:

- Improved mobility and less stress on your joints
- Lowered risk of osteoarthritis
- Greater sense of well-being
- More energy
- Improved mood
- Positive self-image
- Lowered risk of many chronic diseases like some types of cancer, cardiovascular disease, and diabetes
- Decreased levels of inflammation in the body
- Lower blood pressure
- Lower cholesterol
- Better sleep, and in those with sleep apnea (a sleep disorder commonly diagnosed in those with excess weight) improvements and sometimes resolution of the condition

More Than Just Calories and Diet

Even modest weight loss can decrease insulin resistance and improve control. But calorie reduction alone as a weight loss strategy rarely leads to long-term weight control. The three main components of a sound weight loss program include eating a healthy diet (described in Chapter 3), regular physical activity (described in Chapter 4), and behavior modification (described in this chapter).

Behavior Modification

Behavior modification can make all the difference between knowing what to do and actually doing it. Some main principles of behavior modification for weight management include:

1. **Self-monitoring.** Keeping a diary of your weight loss progress and diet can help you become familiar with the things that trigger weight gain and slipups for you, and make you much less likely to fall prey to them the next time around. It helps you see what works for you and what doesn't. It also provides detailed information for your dietitian and doctor to use when creating treatment plans.
2. **Goal setting and shaping.** Deciding upon and setting small goals in the short term can help set you up for long-term success. Meeting your goals and building on them incrementally can be a great motivator to continue to move forward.
3. **Stimulus control.** Identifying triggers that create barriers and setbacks to achieving your weight loss goals is key so that you can prevent them and correct them.
4. **Stress management.** Stress, depression, and mood issues can create large roadblocks to achieving your goals. It is important to find techniques to manage

stress and identify and deal with (in some cases get medical treatment) any mood disorders that you may be experiencing.

5. **Social support.** It can be tough to lose weight all on your own. Creating a support network of family, friends, medical professionals, and even support groups can help give you that extra encouragement you need, as well as help with problem-solving and staying positive through your challenges.

Emotional Eating

Emotional eating is defined as eating in response to emotional triggers such as stress or negative emotions. It can occur in response to dieting or independently on its own due to other factors such as history of emotional trauma, negative life events, and sleep deprivation. Emotional eating is often used as a way to cope with negative feelings, or as a distraction to try to avoid them. During an emotional eating episode it is common to turn to comfort foods that are high in sugar, salt, and fat, which leads to feelings of guilt, which then triggers more emotional eating, becoming an unhealthy cycle.

If you think that you may have problems with emotional eating, especially if it is repeated and out of control, it is important to get help. The best thing you can do is be honest with yourself that there is a problem. There is no shame in admitting and trying to get better. Working with a behavioral therapist and dietitian can help you identify triggers, process your feelings, and develop positive nonfood coping mechanisms, and it can ensure that you have a meal plan that is not too strict, leading to feelings of deprivation that may put you at risk for emotional eating to begin with.

alert

Be aware of the signs of emotional eating. Common signs of emotional eating behavior are sudden onset of intense need to eat (namely unhealthy foods), mindless eating of often large quantities of food, not feeling satisfied despite eating a lot of calories, and feelings of guilt or shame after an episode of eating.

First Steps in Your Weight Loss Journey

To successfully lose weight it is crucial to form a plan. And while it can be difficult to decipher all the information about weight loss out there, the coming chapters in this book are full of healthy eating, exercise, and other important lifestyle recommendations. It is also important to talk with your medical team and a dietitian to develop a specific, individualized weight loss program that incorporates a meal plan, physical activity, and behavior modification to address insulin resistance.

Here are some additional tips:

- Plan regular visits with your team to set goals, weigh in, evaluate progress, and help deal with setbacks.

- Come prepared to medical and dietitian visits with a list of questions and issues and a food diary to maximize your time together and to help them help you.
- Don't be afraid to speak up if you have concerns: The more you share, the better your team can work with you to assist you in succeeding.

Set Realistic Expectations

Expecting that you will lose weight quickly is not realistic or long-lasting. Losing a half pound to one pound a week over a period of time will go much further in helping you achieve results.

---

question

Do weight loss supplements work?

It may be tempting to buy the latest gimmick that promises quick and easy weight loss, but don't do it. Most weight loss supplements are not proven by sound research, are not regulated by the Food and Drug Administration (FDA), and may have ingredients that can interact with medications you are taking or harm your body in general. For some diets, a reputable vitamin and mineral supplement may be beneficial. Always consult with your doctor and dietitian before starting any sort of supplement.

Realize that any weight loss is a good thing in the end. Instead of focusing on a specific weight number on the scale, use positive observations to stay on track. Clothing that fits better or an increased energy level are good ways to gauge your progress. Keep things in perspective, and remind yourself that whatever amount of weight you lose will benefit your blood sugar control and overall health.

Scale Back on Weighing

Don't weigh yourself obsessively. Remember weight loss is not a quick process. Once a week—at the same time of day—is all you need to monitor your progress. Set a regular time to weigh yourself weekly. Keep this in mind:

1. **Be consistent about when and how you weigh yourself.** Weight can vary daily due to fluid shifts, hormones, time of day taken, and clothing worn. It is best to weigh yourself in the same manner each time. First thing in the morning after using the restroom and without clothes is most accurate.
2. **Try to rely more on the way you feel.** If the scale tells you you're losing weight more slowly than you'd like, but you're feeling energetic and positive about your weight loss efforts, then you're heading in the right direction.

Your body—and your progress—are more than numbers on that scale. Applaud your victories, and keep up the hard work.

Your Action Plan

By now you understand the potential consequences of untreated insulin resistance and
excess weight. It is important to develop an
action plan to manage and, with some work
on your part, reverse insulin resistance and
maintain a healthy weight. There are multiple important components to your action
plan based on healthy habits and making key
changes that will be outlined in the next few
chapters:

- Create a sensible eating plan—modify
  your dietary habits
- Get moving and engage in regular
  physical activity
- Make other important lifestyle
  adjustments such as managing stress,
  getting enough sleep, including a social
  support system, and developing good
  problem-solving skills

Once you have made a personal action
plan, you can use the 10-week plan for reversing insulin resistance, recipes, and other tools
in this book to help you get started and stay
on track!

CHAPTER 3

A Sensible Plan for Modifying Your Eating Habits

While there is no magic diet that will suddenly improve insulin resistance or any other health concern, there is an optimal way for people to eat. Consuming more whole, unprocessed foods; increasing the amounts of plant foods; and reducing the amount of fast foods and animal foods all lead to improvements in weight, blood sugar, cholesterol, and other health outcomes.

You may think that having insulin resistance means you will have to give up everything you like to eat, but nothing could be further from the truth! With the help of this chapter, and advice of a registered dietitian, you can adopt healthy eating habits that fit into your lifestyle. Realize that you won't be able to change your eating habits overnight. It is much easier to adopt the approach of taking small steps every day. Over time, you can make significant changes toward improving your health and decreasing insulin resistance.

Eating Styles

Certain patterns of eating, what is often referred to as a *diet*, have extensive research suggesting they are the most healthful for weight reduction and improvements in insulin sensitivity. These eating patterns include the Mediterranean, DASH, and vegetarian diets. They also happen to be the diets that come out on top for heart health, blood sugar control, and reducing cancer risk.

Based on the diets of Mediterranean countries like Greece and Italy, the Mediterranean diet is high in vegetables, fruits, whole grains, beans, nuts and seeds, and olive oil. It also includes moderate amounts of fish, poultry, and dairy products. Red meats and processed foods and sugars are limited. The diet was originally looked at for the low incidence of chronic disease and in particular heart disease in the countries surrounding the Mediterranean Sea, and newer research suggests the Mediterranean diet is linked to lower BMI and waist circumference. In a study comparing patients' adherence to the Mediterranean diet, DASH diet, and American Heart Association diet recommendations, those closest to the Mediterranean diet had the best insulin markers. The PREDIMED study, a randomized, clinical study of cardiovascular risk, published by PREDIMED Study Investigators in 2013, found that the Mediterranean diet improved insulin sensitivity when compared to the control diet.

The DASH (Dietary Approach to Stop Hypertension) diet focuses on lots of whole grains, fruits, vegetables, and low-fat dairy products. It also includes some fish, legumes, and poultry, as well as moderate amounts of nuts and seeds. An initial study in 1997 by the DASH Collaborative Research Group had a group of adults follow a typical American diet for 3 weeks, then assigned them to 8 weeks of either a diet higher in fruits and vegetables or one with more fruits, vegetables, low-fat dairy, and lower saturated and total fat. Both groups improved blood pressure, but the group with the added low-fat dairy and controlled fat intake made greater improvements. Since then, at least two studies in women with PCOS have seen improvements in insulin sensitivity and reduction in insulin levels when a DASH diet is followed, compared with a similar diet with fewer whole plant foods and low-fat dairy items.

The DASH diet suggests the following amounts:

- Whole grains: 6–8 daily servings
- Lean meats or fish: 6 or fewer daily servings
- Vegetables: 4–5 daily servings
- Fruits: 4–5 daily servings
- Lean dairy products: 2–3 daily servings
- Fats and oils: 2–3 or fewer daily servings
- Nuts, seeds, or legumes: 4–5 weekly servings
- Sweets and added sugars: 5 or fewer weekly servings

Vegetarian diets have gained in popularity due to interest in the overall health benefits as well as the benefits to the planet. Many observational, population-based studies, as well as randomized studies, show vegetarian eating as the best to manage weight and blood sugar. The Adventist Health Study, ongoing research out of Loma Linda University in California, has identified a difference of, on average, 30 pounds between vegans and nonvegetarians of the same age and height. A more recent study looked at a group of 35- to 70-year-olds in New Zealand. One group was instructed to follow a low-fat, plant-based diet with no calorie restriction, and the controls continued their diet as usual. End points of BMI and cholesterol reduction were more significant in the plant-based diet participants, and even at long-term follow-up points, 12 months out from the study, risk factor reduction was maintained.

One can choose whether to add 0–2 servings a day of dairy and eggs to their vegetarian diet depending on personal goals and beliefs. If you choose not to eat fish, then including plant sources of omega-3 fats daily is encouraged; try flax, walnuts, chia seeds, canola oil, or an algae-based omega-3 supplement. If you decide to stay on an exclusively plant-based diet, then meet with a registered dietitian to determine if you need any additional supplementation, such as vitamin B_{12}.

What the Mediterranean, DASH, and vegetarian diets share is a focus on less processed, whole plant foods, with a reduction in animal foods. Whole grains, vegetables, fruits, beans, nuts, and seeds make up the majority of these diets, balanced out with seafood, plant-based fat sources such as avocado and olive oil, with limited low-fat dairy, eggs, and occasional meat. All of these foods are made up of macronutrients, the major nutrients your body needs to supply energy, build muscle, maintain your immune system, and carry out all of your bodily functions.

question

What are the different types of vegetarian diets?

Vegetarian diets generally don't include meat, poultry, or fish, yet vegetarian diets can vary in what foods they include and exclude. Lacto-vegetarian diets exclude meat, fish, poultry, and eggs, along with foods that contain them. They do include dairy products, such as milk, cheese, yogurt, and butter. Ovo-vegetarian diets exclude meat, poultry, seafood, and dairy products, yet they allow eggs. Lacto-ovo vegetarian diets exclude meat, fish, and poultry, but include dairy products and eggs. Pescatarian diets exclude meat and poultry, dairy, and eggs, but allow fish.

Carbohydrates and Fiber

Carbohydrates, or carbs, are your body's primary source of glucose, and glucose is your cellular fuel. The body begins to convert carbs almost entirely into glucose shortly after carb-containing foods are eaten. Insulin helps to "unlock" the cells to move the glucose from the bloodstream into the cells for energy. If you have insufficient insulin production or your body is resistant to insulin, consuming too many carbs can cause blood sugar to rise. Having insulin resistance does not mean you must cut out carbs from your diet, but it does mean that making the best carb food choices and determining the appropriate portion size is important to understand.

All foods that contain starches and/or sugars—including fruits, vegetables, milk, yogurt, breads, grains, beans, and pasta—contain carbs. Simple carbs include sugars, sweets, juices, and fruits. Complex carbs include all types of grain products and starchy vegetables such as potatoes and corn. The only whole foods that are virtually carb-free are protein-rich meats, poultry, and fish (when prepared without additional ingredients such as breading and marinades), and fats such as cooking oils and butter.

Avoiding all carb-containing foods is both impossible and unadvisable: Your body needs the fiber, important micronutrients, prebiotics (nutrients that promote growth of beneficial gut bacteria), and plant-based phytochemicals contained in these foods. But you also need to learn the basics of assessing the quantity and quality of carbs in your food, how your body reacts to them, and how to make smart carb choices based on this information.

For meal planning purposes, carbs are put into five categories. The five groups and example servings are as follows:

1. **Starches/Starchy Vegetables:** ⅓ cup cooked rice or pasta, 1 slice of bread, ½ cup cooked oatmeal, ½ cup corn or peas, 1 cup butternut squash.

2. **Fruits:** 1 whole piece of fruit (size of tennis ball) like an orange or apple, 1 cup cubed fruit, ¾ cup berries.
3. **Milk/Yogurt:** 1 cup milk or 6 ounces light yogurt.
4. **Nonstarchy Vegetables:** 1 cup raw vegetables or ½ cup cooked.
5. **"Other" Carbs:** 2 small cookies, ½ cup pudding.

At one time, nutritionists believed that people with diabetes should avoid simple sugars (monosaccharides and disaccharides) and eat foods that contain complex carbs instead. This recommendation was founded on the mistaken belief that simple sugars would raise glucose levels faster and more dramatically across the board. But it's now known that, gram for gram, the complex carbs found in breads, cereals, potatoes, vegetables, and other foods raise blood sugar approximately the same amount as do simple sugars like honey, fructose, or table sugar.

How Many Carbs and What Types Can I Eat?

The precise amount of carbs to include in your diet varies based on your individual energy needs. According to the MyPlate US Department of Agriculture (USDA) guidelines, half your plate should be fruits and vegetables and a quarter whole grains per meal, whereas the DASH diet recommends 4–5 servings of vegetables and 4–5 servings of fruit per day, along with 7–8 daily grain servings.

fact

If a whole-grain ingredient is not listed as the first ingredient, the item may contain only a small portion of whole grains. One way to find a whole-grain product is to look for one of three Whole Grain Stamps. A 100% Stamp label means all grain ingredients are whole grain, with a minimum of 16 grams per serving. The 50%+ Stamp indicates half the grain ingredients are whole grain, with a minimum of 8 grams per serving. A Basic Stamp means at least 8 grams are whole grain but there may also be some refined grain.

Your diet should be individualized depending on your weight, activity level, medications, and medical history.

Why Fiber Is Important

Fiber is considered a carb, but since the body cannot digest most of the fiber, it does not effectively contribute to a rise in blood sugar levels. Fiber is critical to the health of the digestive tract, not only in keeping you regular, but also feeding the bacteria that work as an important mediator of tissue health in the large intestine.

In addition, fiber improves satiety, or the feeling of fullness you get when eating. Fiber delays stomach emptying, helping people to stay fuller longer, and in those people with insulin resistance, pre-diabetes, or type 2 diabetes who are also overweight, the satiety that fiber provides can be a useful tool for achieving both weight loss and blood sugar control.

There are two types of fiber found in foods: soluble and insoluble. It's important to include foods containing both types of fiber in your daily eating plan.

SOLUBLE FIBER

Soluble fiber dissolves and then swells when it's put into water. This type of fiber helps keep blood sugar levels stable by slowing down the rate of glucose absorption into the bloodstream. Soluble fiber absorbs the excess intestinal bile acids that help to form cholesterol, so in turn it helps lower blood cholesterol levels as well. Beans, fruit, barley, and oats are especially good sources of soluble fiber.

INSOLUBLE FIBER

Insoluble fiber does not dissolve in water and is not broken down by bacteria, and it passes through the body relatively unchanged. Insoluble fiber is essential for preventing constipation and colon health by helping to maintain regularity. Vegetables, whole-grain foods, and fruit are all good sources of insoluble fiber.

HOW MUCH FIBER SHOULD I EAT?

Some studies have shown an improved weight loss and glucose- and lipid-lowering benefit with fiber intake of up to 50 grams daily. Recent studies into weight management and the effects on fiber intake show an important relationship. One 6-month study

conducted in 2019, led by Derek Miketinas, found a connection between an increase of 4 grams of fiber a day and a 3-pound greater weight loss.

> **essential**
>
> The consumption of fiber without adequate fluid intake can lead to constipation. As you slowly increase your intake of higher-fiber foods, such as whole-grain breads, beans, fruits, and vegetables, slowly increase your water intake as well. Increasing fiber intake slowly can also help to ease any bloating or other unwanted gastrointestinal distress.

The American Diabetes Association (ADA) recommends a daily fiber intake of at least 14 grams per 1,000 calories. Talk to your doctor and dietitian about what level of fiber in your diet is right for you.

Sugar

The no-sugar myth is probably one of the biggest misconceptions about diet and insulin resistance and blood sugar control. The reality is that it isn't sugar specifically that raises blood glucose levels—it's any food that contains carbs, including honey, fruit, milk, bread, and vegetables. Whether it's a spoonful of sugar, a bagel, or a banana, it will cause blood sugar levels to rise.

There is plenty of evidence linking excess sugar, whether from sodas, juice, or processed foods, to weight gain, while whole, unprocessed sugar-containing foods like fruit are linked with weight loss and improved health. Moderation in added sugar intake is important in any diet. The American Heart Association (AHA) recommends limiting the amount of added sugars you consume to no more than 100 calories per day (about 6 teaspoons of sugar) for women and no more than 150 calories per day (about 9 teaspoons) for men.

Sugar Substitutes

Sugar substitutes are never mandatory when you have insulin resistance, but they can offer options to those who wish to use them. Using a sugar substitute in a recipe can slash sugar content and a significant number of calories.

When using sugar substitutes in baking, keep in mind that sweetness is being added to the food, but other traits unique to a baked product (volume, texture, golden-brown color) may be altered.

---

alert

Don't be misled by a "sugar-free" label. Foods containing stevia, polyols, and/ or artificial sweeteners may still contain carbs and calories that should be figured into your meal plan. Read the nutrition facts on the label to get the full story.

Sugar Alcohols

A sugar alcohol is a monosaccharide that has been chemically transformed into its alcohol form. Several naturally occurring sugar alcohols (also called *polyols*) are available, including sorbitol, mannitol, xylitol, lactitol, maltitol, isomalt, erythritol, and hydrogenated starch hydrolysates. Because they are not completely absorbed in the gastrointestinal tract, they don't cause much of a rise in blood glucose levels, which is why people find them desirable. Polyols are frequently used as sweeteners and bulking agents in processed foods marketed as sugar-free. It is important not to overdo it with your intake of sugar alcohols because some people find that they have a laxative effect, causing diarrhea and/or gas.

Alternative Sweeteners

The sweeteners sucralose, saccharin, aspartame, and stevia are all approved by the FDA. They vary in taste, uses, and suitability for cooking or baking. Keep in mind that these sweeteners are processed foods and, with the exception of stevia, not natural, so it is best to consume them in moderation.

Fats and Cholesterol

Fat insulates the body and supplies energy when no carb sources are available. It also enables the body to absorb and process the fat-soluble vitamins A, D, E, and K. Some types of fat may increase the risk of atherosclerosis, which is the buildup of fat, cholesterol, and other substances in the artery walls, collectively referred to as plaque. Atherosclerosis can restrict blood flow. And since fats are higher in calories than the other macronutrients, too much fat can lead to weight gain.

Fats can be confusing to many people when they first start learning about the dietary management of insulin resistance. The off-target message that "all fat is bad" became entrenched in popular dietary culture in the 1990s, turning fat-free food production into a multimillion-dollar industry. While some fats are bad for you in excess, others can help improve your cholesterol profile. Here are the basic dietary fats:

- **Saturated fats.** These are solid fats found in meat and dairy products and vegetable oils. Too much saturated fat in the diet may be associated with high LDL (bad) cholesterol levels. However, research is conflicting as to whether dietary saturated fat actually increases your risk of heart disease, and recent studies dispute this claim.
- **Unsaturated fats.** These are found in plants, as well as fish and seafood. They include polyunsaturated fats (e.g., safflower oil, fish, and walnuts) and monounsaturated fats (e.g., olive oil, nuts, and avocado). These types of fats— polyunsaturated, in particular—have been shown to be effective in reducing total and LDL (bad) cholesterol levels.

- **Trans fats/hydrogenated fats.** These include trans unsaturated fatty acids or unsaturated liquid fats that have been processed into a more saturated and solid form by adding hydrogen. They are often found in processed baked goods and commercial fried foods and may be called *partially hydrogenated* or *hydrogenated fats*. Trans-fatty acids can raise LDL (bad) cholesterol and lower HDL (good) cholesterol, and you should limit your consumption or avoid them altogether.
- **Omega "essential" fatty acids.** These are types of polyunsaturated fat, which have heart-protective benefits and lower both triglyceride levels and blood pressure; they are found in fish and fish oils and certain seeds and nuts and their oils (e.g., flaxseed, canola, soybean, and walnut). Linolenic, alpha-linolenic, eicosapentaenoic, and docosahexaenoic acids are all essential fatty acids.
- **Dietary cholesterol.** This is present in food that comes from animals, including poultry, fish, eggs, meats, and dairy products. Research shows that dietary cholesterol does not make a significant contribution to atherosclerosis in comparison to saturated and trans fats.

How Much Fat Can I Eat?

The National Academy of Medicine has defined an acceptable amount of total fat for all adults to be 20–35 percent of total calorie intake. The type of fat is more important than the total amount consumed, so the goal is to have 10 percent or less of daily calories come from saturated fats, and trans-fat intake should be limited as much as possible. Cholesterol intake should be less than 200 milligrams per day. The ADA also recommends 2 or more servings of fish weekly for the cardioprotective benefits of omega-3 fatty acids. Examples of fat servings would be 1 teaspoon of butter or margarine, ⅛ of a medium avocado, or 1 tablespoon of salad dressing or oil.

Including healthy plant-based fats in small portions can help with satiety and add flavor and healthy nutrients, as well as provide some protective benefits as far as insulin resistance, pre-diabetes, diabetes, and heart disease are concerned. When it comes to weight loss, research shows that reducing fat intake, and increasing lean protein, fruits, and vegetables, leads to more weight reduction. When cooking or adding fat to meals, try to have just a dab of healthy fat.

Lean Proteins

Proteins are chains of amino acids responsible for cell growth and maintenance and are found in virtually every part of the body. Protein in foods from animal sources (meat, poultry, fish, and dairy), as well as soy and hemp, are called *complete proteins* because they contain all the essential amino acids necessary for building and maintaining cells. Protein in other plant-based foods such as grains, beans, fruit, and vegetables are called

incomplete proteins because they contain only partial groups of these amino acids. Eating a variety of different incomplete plant-based proteins can help form complete proteins in your diet. If you are a vegetarian or vegan and have insulin resistance, a dietitian with experience in vegetarian menu planning can advise you on appropriate protein consumption choices.

How Much Protein Should I Eat?

Protein intake goals should be individualized, but it is recommended that people—especially those with insulin resistance—should have 15–20 percent of their total daily calories from protein. Some research has suggested that higher protein diets with 20–30 percent of daily calories from protein may be beneficial to help with feeling full longer. When it comes to weight loss and insulin resistance, choosing more plant proteins and having regular fish intake to meet protein needs is the best choice. People with impaired kidney function, or nephropathy, may need to avoid a high-protein diet because damaged kidneys cannot filter protein efficiently from the bloodstream. If you have kidney problems, talk to your doctor and dietitian about an appropriate level of protein for your diet. Examples of protein servings would be 3–5 ounces of chicken, fish, pork, or red meat, and ½ cup tofu or beans.

The Balance of Sodium and Fluid Intake

In moderate amounts, dietary sodium, or sodium chloride (salt), is not harmful. In fact, this mineral helps to maintain a healthy electrolyte balance and works in tandem with potassium to regulate the balance of acidic and basic substances in the blood, as well as heart function, nerve impulses, and muscle contractions. People with high blood pressure need to be cautious about having too much sodium in their daily diet. The 1997 DASH diet study found that limiting dietary sodium is associated with a substantial reduction in blood pressure in adults with hypertension. There is also some evidence that higher-sodium diets affect hormone levels associated with abdominal fat storage, in turn affecting insulin resistance.

How Much Sodium Should I Eat?

The recommended daily sodium intake is 2,300 milligrams, equivalent to a teaspoon of sodium chloride, or table salt, per the American Heart Association. The average American, however, consumes more than twice that much. Processed and fast foods such as pizza, burgers, and snack foods are the major culprits. Watch out for added sodium in condiments, as well as packaged and canned foods. Some people with hypertension may benefit from an even bigger cut in dietary salt intake. Studies have shown that reducing sodium intake to 1,500 milligrams daily reduces blood pressure significantly when it is part of the DASH diet.

Think about What You Drink

You may already know that it's important to drink plenty of fluids throughout the day, but you also need to pay attention to the quality of your fluids, not just the quantity. Water is your best bet because it hydrates you simply, without anything added. Focus on consuming water as your main source of hydration to cut calories, sugar, and additives. Try to keep what you drink as simple as possible.

What about Alcohol?

When it comes to alcohol and your health, the optimal word is always *moderation*. Consider the facts about alcohol and decide whether including alcohol on a moderate basis fits into your insulin resistance management plan. Alcohol does not provide any essential nutrients, but it is a source of calories. If you drink and are having difficulty losing weight, do not overlook the calories that alcohol adds to your overall intake. Alcohol can also impact blood lipid levels and elevate triglycerides. Both health issues may already be a source of concern for you.

It is perfectly okay to add a small amount of alcohol in certain recipes. A bit of wine or flavored liqueur can enhance the flavor of the food and can be incorporated as a low-fat cooking ingredient or marinade. When cooked, the alcohol content diminishes, but the flavor remains.

Reducing Calories

A calorie (a.k.a. *kilocalorie*) is defined as the amount of energy required to raise the temperature of 1 gram of water by 1°C. Simply put, it is a unit of energy your body uses as fuel. The three main macronutrients, or sources of calories, are carbs, proteins, and fats. Carbs and proteins each provide 4 calories per gram, whereas fats provide 9 calories per gram. Alcohol provides 7 calories per gram. Foods tend to be mixtures of carbs, proteins, and fats; each food has its own unique calorie value that you find on nutrition labels and in food charts. Keep in mind that when you are on a particular calorie budget for weight loss, you want to consume foods that are nutrient-dense, meaning they have the most nutrients, like healthy carbs, proteins, fats, fiber, vitamins, and minerals, for the lowest number of calories they contain.

What Should My Caloric Intake Be?

Your ideal calorie intake is based on your activity level, gender, age, and other factors. Reducing calorie intake is one component of an effective weight reduction program, so it is also an important consideration in the dietary management of insulin resistance.

The estimated amounts of daily calorie intake based on gender, age, and activity levels from the USDA's *2015–2020 Dietary Guidelines for Americans* can be found at https://health.gov/dietaryguidelines/2015/guidelines/appendix-2/. These are general guidelines for weight maintenance, not weight loss. The ADA suggests a lifestyle program with a diet approach of reduced calories (500–750 fewer calories than the USDA guidelines listed for weight maintenance), or approximately 1,200–1,500 calories a day for women and 1,500–1,800 calories a day for men. These guidelines are general, so an important part of this approach involves education and support via meeting with a registered dietitian regularly. You can work together to decide upon your calorie goal and get an individualized meal plan that will be helpful to your efforts to lose weight. Focus on making changes for the long term that you can live with and allow you to eat a variety of foods you enjoy.

Maintaining a Healthy Diet

As you compare your eating style to the different well-researched, healthy approaches, you can use the following strategies to continue on and refine your week-to-week actions until you reach your goal.

Practice Portion Control

It's a good idea to measure most foods and beverages you consume until you get a feel for portion sizes. That way you are less likely to overdo it, which can lead to higher blood sugars and excess weight.

The only tools you really need to measure your portions are a simple and inexpensive gram scale, dry and liquid measuring cups, and measuring spoons.

Stick To a Consistent Schedule

It is important to fuel yourself adequately throughout the day. Excess hunger can lead to overeating, not to mention making you feel downright cranky, and it can work against your health goals. There is research that those who eat breakfast daily make healthier food choices and control their weight better.

Find a schedule that works for you, whether you restrict your eating to 8 hours, or eat two meals, three meals, or six meals a day. The goals are to manage hunger, stay within calorie needs, and choose healthy, unprocessed foods.

Choose Carbs Wisely

Starches provide the body with energy. Keep starch portions to a quarter of your plate, and choose whole-grain varieties, such as whole wheat, oats, and quinoa, that are high in fiber. Starchy vegetables are also great choices. Corn on the cob, peas, sweet potatoes, and butternut squash provide loads of fiber, vitamins, and minerals. The best way to get more whole grains and starchy vegetables in your meals is to substitute refined products with whole-grain or vegetable options. Gradually start replacing the refined grains in your kitchen cabinets with whole-grain foods and consume moderate portions.

Fill Up on Nonstarchy Vegetables

Pile half your plate with raw and/or cooked vegetables to achieve satiety and keep your nutrient and fiber intake high and your calories and fat intake low. There are a lot of great ways to increase the portions of vegetables in your meals. Be creative to get in plenty of vegetables daily. For example, add spinach, tomato, mushrooms, and more to your breakfast omelet or egg scramble; include a large salad with each dinner; toss mushrooms or onions into your pasta sauce; or blend spinach, beets, or carrots into a smoothie.

Choose Moderate Amounts of Low-Fat Dairy

Both the ADA and the USDA recommend consuming low-fat rather than full-fat dairy products. Traditionally, this recommendation has been based on the presumed link between saturated fat and heart disease, but more research is being conducted regularly to see if we really need to shy away entirely from saturated fat. For now, get in the habit of limiting full-fat dairy to small amounts and know that low-fat dairy products such as cheese, cottage cheese, yogurt, and milk are lower in fat and calories. They help with satiety, and they are good sources of calcium for bone health, as well as protein for muscle mass.

Feast on Fruits in Their Natural Form

When it comes to fruit, whole and fresh is the best choice. That way you get all the nutrients and fiber without added sugar. Fruits contain natural sugars (fructose) that raise blood sugar levels, yet they also have fiber to help moderate that effect. It's all about choosing fresh fruit and watching portions.

Pick Protein Wisely

The good news is, when prepared without sauces or breading, lower-fat cuts of meat, poultry, and fish are chock-full of protein that will help keep you full for weight control. Plant protein sources, like beans, have the added benefit of being low-fat and full of fiber. Aim to include a good source of protein at each meal.

Add Small Portions of Healthy Fats

Remember to keep portions of fat small and to choose healthy, plant-based unsaturated fats, as well as aim for 2 or more servings of fish weekly for the cardioprotective benefits of omega-3 fatty acids.

Reduce Sodium Intake

There are still plenty of ways you can spice things up and flavor your food that don't involve salt. Try low-sodium condiments and flavorings like fresh basil, lemon, pepper, garlic, mustard, salsa, vinegars, and commercial herb blends to season food instead of using salt.

Focus On Healthy Fluids

Water is your best choice when it comes to filling your glass. Avoid sodas, fruit juices, smoothies, and sweetened coffee drinks.

Don't sabotage your menu plan by consuming empty calories and sugar. Instead:

- Add a squeeze of lemon or lime to your water
- Add basil, mint, berries, citrus, or cucumber to sparkling water
- Go for decaffeinated black tea or coffee with a little low-fat or plant-based milk, and use vanilla extract and cinnamon for added flavor

Make Healthy Choices on a Budget

You don't have to spend tons of money to stick to a sensible meal plan for your insulin resistance. There are many ways to choose a variety of healthy foods that still fit your budget, including:

- Buying whole grains and other staples in bulk
- Choosing generic brands or store-brand versions of popular whole-grain cereals and breads

- Making your own homemade baked goods
- Shopping for fruits and vegetables that are in season
- Buying whole-leaf greens instead of bagged salads
- Buying milk, yogurt, cheese, cottage cheese, eggs, and fresh meats on sale weekly

Don't be afraid to clip coupons and shop around: Eating right doesn't have to be expensive!

Shop Smart

Being prepared and in the right frame of mind can make all the difference when you are shopping for food. Never go to the grocery store hungry, as this can increase the temptation to buy less-healthy food. Also, take the time to plan ahead before you grocery shop. Make a list of foods that fit your meal plan so you can arrive prepared and maximize your time while in the store.

Dine Out Within Your Meal Plan

Keep it clean and simple when eating out. Planning ahead and making smart substitutions and good menu choices can help you keep within the scope of your meal plan. Remember to use the plate method (plate = ¼ protein, ¼ starch, and ½ nonstarchy vegetables) when making food choices. Skip the bread basket or chips, and start with a salad or broth-based soup instead. Also, request all condiments be served on the side.

The best restaurant menu picks include dishes prepared with tomato sauces rather than cream sauces; grilled, poached, or broiled fish or poultry dishes; grilled or broiled meats served without gravies or sauces; vegetables that have been steamed or lightly sautéed or grilled; high-fiber starches such as brown rice, whole-wheat pasta, or baked potato with the skin (but keep portions to a quarter of the plate); broth-based soups instead of cream soups; and salads with dressing on the side and minus the extras such as cheese and croutons.

For dessert, order a single item for the table and just have a bite or two, order fruit, or enjoy a sugar-free hard candy or a small healthy dessert within your meal plan waiting for you at home.

Snack Sensibly

Snacks are a great way to keep you energized and to prevent excess hunger, as well as overeating at mealtimes, but don't get sabotaged by a snack attack gone haywire. Too much snacking, particularly eating the wrong foods, can send your weight out of control. Choosing the right snacks to have between meals can make all the difference in helping you along with your meal plan. It can be helpful to consume snacks that are high in fiber, as well as mini combos of protein and fat to help satisfy you and keep your blood sugar more stable until the next mealtime.

Investigate Ingredients Lists

Keep it simple and natural as far as your meal plan is concerned. Steer clear of processed foods as often as you can; a long list of ingredients should be a red flag. Cut down on packaged foods that may have additives such as sugar and salt, not to mention tons of stabilizers and chemicals that you may not even be able to pronounce. You can take the guesswork out of food choices by choosing whole and natural foods like fresh fruits and vegetables; whole-grain staples like oatmeal, brown rice, and corn tortillas; and fresh meats and poultry; along with nuts and natural nut butters, to name a few examples. Try to eat more fresh food that you can prepare yourself at home.

Learn the Food Label Lingo

Take time to read and understand labels so you get to know your food better. Focus on key components on the label such as serving size, amount of nutrients per serving, and the ingredients list:

1. **Serving size.** Each label must identify the size of a serving. The nutritional information listed on a label is based on 1 serving of the food.
2. **Amount per serving.** Each package identifies the quantities of nutrients and food constituents from 1 serving.
3. **Percent daily value.** This indicates how much of a specific nutrient a serving of food contains in comparison to an average 2,000-calorie diet.

4. **Ingredients list.** This is a listing of the ingredients in a food in descending order of predominance and weight.

You may see that there are several parts to the carb section of the nutrition label. The total carb number represents the amount of carb grams found in a food. Beneath the total carb line are other carb listings: fiber, sugars, added sugars, and, sometimes, sugar alcohols.

Cook Creatively to Keep Healthy

There are many ways to prepare foods that not only preserve nutrients and good taste but also minimize the use of sugar, salt, and fat. A little creativity with spices, herbs, or combining foods together in unconventional ways makes food more flavorful without the addition of extra fat, sodium, or calories. Preparing your foods in healthy ways can ensure that your home-cooked meals are in accordance with your meal plan.

Stir-frying, broiling, and slow cooking are examples of techniques that are time-saving and result in more healthful food. Instant Pots® and air fryers have also become popular options for easier meals. Air frying also allows you to enjoy the crunch and flavor of fried foods, without the high-carb, high-calorie breading and high-fat oil.

Bake Homemade to Help Lower Sugar and Fat

Baking at home helps you control the sugar, fat, and calories to help your favorite recipes coincide with healthy eating to reduce insulin resistance. When adjusting the sugar content, it's best to start with a smaller reduction (25 percent) and gradually decrease the amount each time you make that dish. Be sure to note whether the properties of the food have any significant or undesirable changes, then adjust as needed. To replace fat, but not volume, try using plain yogurt, applesauce, mashed ripe banana, or other puréed fruit for half of the oil or shortening called for in a recipe.

Plan to Treat Yourself Once in a While

Of course, it is difficult to never eat the foods you love. If you decide never to eat a particular food, you may become obsessed with it and end up overeating it when given the opportunity. Lifelong healthy eating is about choices and finding a way to balance all the foods that you enjoy within reason as far as your meal plan is concerned.

Don't deprive yourself of the foods you love; instead, give yourself permission to eat and enjoy them by reserving them for a certain time, and remember portion control. Also, plan to "cheat" by eating lighter at meals before and after your splurge.

Stock Your Pantry and Refrigerator with the Right Foods

Having healthy alternatives available when you are hungry encourages adherence to your meal plan, whereas having high-calorie foods, snacks, and desserts invites temptation. Relying on willpower to stop you from eating irresistible foods will not work if you are faced with these food choices every day. In fact, willpower should not be one of your ongoing strategies to improve your eating habits. Instead, keep yourself in check by stocking your pantry and refrigerator with healthy choices. Check out Appendix B for a list of great healthy options to stock up on.

Eat Mindfully

We are all so busy these days it is too easy to gobble down a meal without knowing how much we've eaten. Make time to focus on your food and enjoy it by taking time out to eat without distractions like the TV or your phone; otherwise it is easy to lose track and decrease the positive control you can have over your eating habits.

Focus on how the food looks, smells, and tastes, and enjoy the different textures as you eat. Pay attention to when you feel full.

Next Steps

Despite an abundance of ways to start eating healthier, it's up to you to determine the most realistic, easy, and enjoyable path for you. Start with one small change at a time, follow up and see how the change worked for you, then move on to the next goal. In the next chapter, you'll pair your dietary changes with some exercise changes to really attack insulin resistance!

CHAPTER 4

Get Moving

Being more active is an important part of your insulin resistance plan. One of the simplest and most effective ways to decrease insulin resistance, manage your weight, cut the risk of cardiovascular disease, and improve overall health and well-being is exercise. Despite these benefits, exercise is a tough sell in an increasingly sedentary world where almost every essential task can be performed online, from the driver's seat, or with a phone call.

Redefining your preconceived notions of exercise, and making it fun, is the best way to ensure that you look forward to exercising instead of finding ways to avoid it. In this chapter, you'll learn about the different types of exercise and ways to incorporate regular exercise into your routine in order to manage insulin resistance. You may be surprised by how many types of activity count as exercise and can be beneficial to your health!

The Importance of Exercise

Everyone should exercise, yet the National Health Interview Survey reveals that less than half of the US adult population gets the recommended 30 minutes of daily physical activity—and 33 percent aren't active at all. Inactivity is thought to be one of the key reasons for the surge of obesity and diabetes in the US, and inactivity and obesity promote insulin resistance. Interestingly, research shows that exercise improves insulin resistance for up to 48–72 hours post-workout, but that as soon as you stop exercising for 3–5 days, the benefits can begin to wane.

The good news is that it's never too late to get moving, and exercise is one of the easiest ways to start controlling your insulin resistance. Remember that just like changes to the foods you eat, the exercise you choose and how and when you do it needs to be sustainable and fit into your lifestyle.

How Exercise Helps Control Insulin Resistance

Regular activity and exercise improves insulin resistance. Lower blood sugar levels are achieved when the glucose in your blood is used for energy during and after exercise; in fact this improvement can be as much as 40 percent above normal. Exercise combats insulin resistance by its positive influences on three major parts of your body:

1. **Muscles.** With increased activity, muscle cells become more sensitive to insulin, allowing for better storage and usage of glucose for energy. Improvements seen in muscle cells come from various changes that take place with exercise, such as the activation of GLUT4, an important glucose transport molecule, and more effective insulin receptors. A reduction in fatty acid storage in muscles through repeated exercise also leads to some of the improvements seen in insulin sensitivity.
2. **Pancreas.** While the beta cells of the pancreas may be overworked with rising insulin resistance, studies looking at regular exercise and weight loss show improvement in beta cell function. Much of the improvement is dose dependent, meaning with more intense, and longer, bouts of exercise, greater achievement in the beta cell function is observed.
3. **Liver.** After exercise, the liver is better at storing extra glucose from food, as glycogen, reducing glucose levels in the blood. Cells in the liver become more sensitive to insulin release, thus preventing the liver from providing excess glucose that the body doesn't need.

While more exercise seems to show greater improvements across all areas related to insulin resistance, studies consistently show that 30 minutes, 3 or more days per week, of "moderate" activity, such as walking, improves blood sugar control and insulin sensitivity. Even research in children shows that when kids achieve greater physical activity levels in school, they have better insulin sensitivity. Playing more, walking, dancing, jumping, using your muscles to move in all different ways, helps the whole body!

Routine exercise is vital to the process of stopping insulin resistance from progressing to pre-diabetes and diabetes, and for improving your overall health.

First Steps in Your Exercise Routine

If this was not initially discussed during conversations about insulin resistance, you should talk to your doctor to make sure that exercise is appropriate for you. In most cases, your doctor will support your desire to start an exercise plan. If you have other health issues in addition to insulin resistance, you and your doctor should discuss the best types of exercise for you.

Be realistic when choosing exercises for yourself. Once your doctor has given you the okay to start, it's time to consider the variables that will help you choose the right type of exercise:

- Consider your physical ability to perform certain activities and choose ones that you can do
- Include activities you enjoy or increase those already performed on a semi-regular basis like taking the dog for a walk, gardening, or even vacuuming
- Think about how much time you have, as an ambitious exercise plan that involves too much time will quickly be abandoned if you lack the time
- If you have not exercised recently, ease into a program that includes short periods to start with
- Consider the resources available to you, such as a gym, workout equipment, pool, or simply a safe route to walk along near your home

When you make plans for exercise and activity, it is important to be honest about your likelihood to maintain the plan. Make sure to plan activities that you will enjoy or do not mind doing. Would you prefer to exercise alone or with the company of a friend or spouse? Will your activity involve being outdoors or indoors? Can you perform the activity outdoors year-round or will you need to find an alternate indoor activity for part of the year? Try to work out any barriers ahead of time that could get in the way of your exercise plan.

question

Do I need to buy a lot of exercise equipment?

Resist the temptation to purchase home exercise equipment until you have tried it out and are sure that you will use it. Many types of home equipment end up at garage sales or just taking up space because the owner stopped using the equipment after a short period of time. Make sure you like the activity enough that you will want to do it often!

Establish Safety

While physical activity can be a great thing for your health, make sure to take the proper precautions to avoid injury or exhaustion. You should:

- Consult with your doctor before beginning an exercise program to obtain medical approval
- Warm up and stretch your muscles for at least 5 minutes before beginning a workout, and do a 5-minute cooldown at the end as well
- Avoid exercising outside in extreme temperatures (superhot or very cold), or consider changing your workout to indoors in these temperatures
- Exercise at an intensity that feels moderate and comfortable; don't overdo it

- Wear breathable, comfortable clothing and sturdy footwear during workouts
- Hydrate adequately before, during, and after your workout
- Get initial instruction about proper form and positioning from an experienced trainer if working out with weights
- Stop activity if you feel any pain, dizziness, difficulty breathing, or chest pain, and let your doctor know if you have experienced any of these symptoms during exercise

Along with regular activity, safety should be a priority in your action plan to conquer insulin resistance.

Feel Good in Your Body

If you are new to exercise, you may find that some forms of movement feel better than others. Comfort is important; certain exercises such as jogging may not be feasible right off the bat, but walking, swimming, and dancing are examples of activities that most people can participate in at an appropriate intensity level. Listen to your body!

It's possible you may not feel mentally or emotionally prepared to join group or team exercises. If you feel uncomfortable amid all the spandex at the local health club, then don't torture yourself—find an environment that you feel better in. Try a walking program, either outside or at home on a treadmill or along with an online video. Buddy up with a friend and motivate each other to reach workout goals. Exercise should make you feel good about yourself. Every step you take is a step toward a healthier you.

Remember that if you have any specific concerns, you should check with your doctor before starting a fitness routine. A referral to an exercise physiologist may be appropriate, particularly if you have other health problems. Other fitness professionals, like certified personal trainers, yoga instructors, and other fitness class instructors, can help you find a good beginning routine and adapt exercises to your ability level.

Make Time for Exercise

Along with safety precautions and a focus on what feels comfortable for your body, your exercise routine should also be planned to fit naturally into your daily schedule. Look at your daily routine, then decide where you can realistically fit in some time for activity. If you have busy days, short periods of time (10–30 minutes) will probably work much better than trying to carve out an hour every day for activity.

fact

As long as you exercise, the time of day you actually do the exercise is the best time! Busy and demanding schedules often get in the way of good intentions. If your schedule is particularly demanding, try making an appointment on your schedule for your exercise time. Remember that any time spent exercising is better than no time.

Start out with small amounts of time one or more times a day. You will likely have more success getting in activity this way.

Optimize Results

If you really want to stop insulin resistance in its tracks, it is important to understand just how important it is to initiate a plan for physical activity. Many people just focus on changing their eating habits. While this is also important, the lack of exercise could prevent you from reaching your goals. Cutting down on food will not be enough to help you lose weight and maintain a lower weight. Physical activity is a key component to your lifestyle plan and must be included at whatever level you are able to accommodate.

If you are someone who never seems able to find the time or energy for exercise, begin to take a serious look at what the barriers are. Once you identify what is getting in your way, plan strategies to help you go around those barriers. Keep your strategies simple and real. Writing down and implementing your strategy is a good way to help you make permanent changes.

Cardio Exercise

The 2018 *Physical Activity Guidelines for Americans* recommends a minimum of 150 minutes of moderate-intensity aerobic exercise weekly. Ideally, no more than 2 days should pass between exercise sessions. With younger and more physically fit individuals, the shorter durations (minimum 75 minutes per week) of vigorous-intensity or interval training may be enough. But ultimately, starting slow and working up to the 150 minutes a week is the way to go. The following are a variety of simple ways you can add aerobic exercise into your routine.

Get Walking

For most people, walking is a good place to begin an exercise program because it is easy and requires no special equipment other than a pair of good walking shoes or sneakers. Brisk walking is considered an aerobic exercise, which means your body is using oxygen. Aerobic exercise increases your heart rate and burns calories. Walking in this manner is considered an effective type of exercise for weight loss. And any extra walking you do throughout the day also adds up, so try walking as a good start to your exercise plan.

If you choose to walk and have not exercised in a long time, you may need to begin by walking at a moderate pace. Walking about three times a week for a period of 10–15 minutes can help ease you into a routine. As you become stronger and gain more endurance, gradually increase your walking time by 5 minutes every 1–2 weeks, until you are able to walk for a full 30 minutes. Once you are comfortable walking for 30 minutes, increase your frequency to four or five times weekly, and gradually pick up the pace to a brisk walk.

Try an Exercise Class

Enrolling in a class at your local gym, fitness center, or recreation center is a great way to try something new, meet others, and get some helpful guidance from an instructor. Incorporate fitness classes to help add variety into your exercise routine to improve your blood sugars and manage weight. Take advantage of all your options. There are so many to choose from these days, such as yoga, Pilates, aerobics, CrossFit, kickboxing, sculpting, water aerobics—you name it! When you find a class you like, check to see if the gym or fitness center offers specials or the option to pay for a block of classes ahead of time. Doing this will often get you a small discount, and it also helps hold you accountable for showing up to multiple sessions in the future.

Many classes incorporate weights or exercises using your own body weight, which can be a great way to get your resistance training under the observation of a skilled instructor.

Intimidated by the thought of doing a class in public? Look into fitness workouts via DVD or online videos. You can try them in the comfort of your own home.

Exercise Intensity

How hard you should push yourself during a workout depends on your level of fitness and your health history. Your doctor can recommend an optimal heart rate target for working out based on those factors. It's very important to get this information from your doctor before starting an exercise program, especially if you have a history of cardio-vascular problems. On average, most people should aim for a target heart rate zone of

50–75 percent of their maximum heart rate. Maximum heart rate is found by subtracting your age from the number 220. So, if you are 40, your maximum heart rate would be 180, and your target heart rate zone would be between 90 and 135 beats per minute.

You should wear a digital or analog watch with a second hand or function to check your heart rate during exercise. To calculate your heart rate, place your fingers at your wrist or neck pulse point and count the number of beats for fifteen seconds. Multiply that number by 4 to get your heart rate. The number you get should be within your target zone. If it's too high, take your intensity down a few notches. If you're exercising below your target zone, pick things up. If you are new to exercise, you should aim for the lower (50 percent) range of your target heart rate. As you become more fit, you can work toward the 75 percent maximum.

Resistance Training and Stretching

In addition to cardio exercise, it is important to incorporate resistance training into your routine, if possible. Resistance training is strength training that works the muscles. Activities such as weightlifting, working with resistance bands, water workouts, and body weight resistance exercises (e.g., push-ups, pull-ups, and squats) are all good forms of resistance training. Studies have shown that increasing muscle mass through strength training reduces insulin resistance and helps to lower blood glucose. Resistance exercises should work all the major muscle groups of the upper body, lower body, and core. If you include strength training, be sure to allow at least 48 hours between sessions so your muscles are able to rest and recover.

essential

Resistance bands can be an inexpensive way to do strength training. They help with coordination, add variety to workouts, and are great for all fitness levels. Resistance bands are color-coded to designate tension level, which can vary from light to heavy. Consider talking with a trainer to determine the right bands for you and the best exercises to perform with them.

For most people, short strength-training sessions two to three times weekly will provide added benefit. If you are new to resistance training, it can be helpful to work with a certified trainer for at least a few sessions to determine the right set of exercises for you and to ensure proper form to get the maximum benefits without risking injury.

Know Your Reps

Using resistance training with varied and increasing repetitions and sets can help you get stronger, not to mention help control your insulin resistance. It is important to become familiar with the amount of repetitions and sets of various exercises that should be completed to get the maximum benefits from your routine in a safe way.

Consulting with a certified trainer can take the guesswork out of resistance training (if you have been approved to start strength training by your physician). When doing resistance training with weights or bands, your initial goal should be to try to complete one to two sets of 10–15 repetitions per set. Get to where you are feeling near fatigue in that muscle when done.

As you get stronger you can progress by using gradually heavier weights/resistance to where you can complete at least 8–10 repetitions per set. You can follow the increase in weight/resistance by increasing the number of sets (for example, instead of doing one to two sets of repetitions, try two to three sets). If you have a history of joint or muscle issues or other health limitations, start with just one set of 10–15 repetitions with a lighter weight, and then progress to 15–20 repetitions before increasing the number of sets.

Make Stretching Part of Your Routine

Stretching is another worthwhile addition to a well-rounded exercise plan because it helps to increase flexibility and prevent injury. Stretch slowly, without bouncing, and only stretch as far as you can without causing any pain. A few minutes of stretching at the beginning and end of an exercise session can make exercise easier and reduce the possibility of injury. Stretching has not been shown to have much impact on insulin resistance, so it should not be substituted for aerobic or resistance activity but rather used as an add-on to your workout.

Take It Slow and Steady When Starting A New Routine

Many people with insulin resistance start exercising for the sole purpose of losing weight. When the pounds don't drop as quickly or as completely as they'd like, some of these people get discouraged and give up. If you take away any message about exercise and insulin resistance, let it be this: Even if you don't lose weight, your investment in exercise is still paying off in reduced heart disease risk and better function of the organs involved in insulin resistance. Also remember that exercise builds muscle, which weighs more than fat. If your clothes fit better, but the pounds don't melt off as much as you'd hoped, you are still ahead of the game. It means you have made changes in the storage of visceral fat, improving the functioning of your major organs like the heart, liver, pancreas, and digestive tract. And exercise simply makes you feel better, both physically and mentally. Your energy level will rise, and the endorphins released by your brain during exercise will boost your sense of well-being and may help fight stress and depression. Don't give up before you really get started. You owe it to yourself to keep going.

Creative Ways to Increase Activity

To create success with starting and maintaining your exercise plan, branch out and find new ways to get exercise and keep it interesting. Varying the routine helps to keep you from getting bored, and it challenges your body in different ways. An exercise plan of walking can be augmented by including strength training and stretching. Your exercise program should be one that you can maintain for life. Make sensible decisions about what you can and will change to increase your activity level. You may realize some of the benefits of exercise early on, but long-lasting results come about with consistency. Think of your exercise program as a work in progress that you are constantly improving and finding new ways to derive health benefits and enjoyment from.

The following are other suggestions for integrating exercise into your daily routine.

Invest In a Pedometer

An excellent way to stay motivated and track your progress is to use a pedometer. A pedometer counts the number of steps you take over the course of a day. Most smartphones have a pedometer built into one of the apps already installed on the phone, or you can download a separate pedometer app. You can also buy a separate pedometer to clip to your belt or waistband. Using a pedometer can be helpful to ensure that you are getting in your daily steps to promote control of your insulin resistance.

Make Your Own Soundtrack

Keep your workouts interesting with some audio entertainment! Listen to the radio, or, better yet, make your own custom playlist to enjoy your favorite tunes while exercising. Moving to the beat helps you stay motivated and keep a moderate intensity to your workout. Another option is to exercise your mind and your body with an audiobook or podcast. You can also try exercising without the music and instead enjoy the sounds of nature around you.

Don't Just Sit There

Research has shown that sitting for prolonged periods of time with no physical activity puts a person at similar health risks to smokers. Move around as often as possible to reduce your risk and break the insulin resistance cycle. Avoid sitting for longer than 30–60 minutes. Stand up, take a bathroom break, go get a glass of water, take a short walk, do some squats, or try a few stretches to re-energize and stay healthy. Set a timer while working, walk around during phone calls, and get up during TV commercials.

Break It Up

If you don't have a full 30- to 60-minute block in your day to work out, try working in 10 minutes of activity several times a day; the benefits will add up. There are many ways you can add in a little bit of activity to your day without making huge demands on your schedule. Find opportunities to walk by arriving at your destination early, parking farther away, and then walking for 10 minutes. Avoid elevators by taking the stairs whenever you can. Go for a 10-minute walk after lunch or dinner. Spend 10 minutes at the beginning and end of each day doing a few strength-training and stretching exercises.

Make Exercise a Chore, Literally

You may not realize it, but many routine household activities such as cleaning, vacuuming, carrying groceries, gardening, and yard work are all forms of physical activity that can help bring down blood sugars and burn calories. Include this type of activity in your daily routine. Use your daily chore list as a way to get in more activity and keep a clean house while you are at it. Some examples of different chores and the calories they burn per 30 minutes include:

- "Light" activity: Sweeping, washing dishes, laundry, and dusting = 90–100 calories each
- "Moderate" activity: Gardening, mowing the lawn, raking leaves, scrubbing floors, vacuuming, washing cars, washing windows, carrying out trash, and shoveling snow or dirt = 130–200 calories each

Essentially, if you do 30 minutes of exercise walking a day, then add in a couple of these chores, you can burn an additional 300 calories a day, helping you achieve the calorie deficit needed for weight loss. So, start tidying up!

Pair Up with an Exercise Buddy…or Two or Three

Working out with a friend, family member, or colleague helps keep activity fun and social and is a great motivator for sticking to your exercise plan. It requires you to plan ahead to schedule your activity, and your partner can hold you accountable to complete it. Plus, you will be amazed at how fast the time goes by during your workout when you are walking and talking with a friend. Being able to support one another is a positive feeling. The more exercise buddies, the merrier to keep things upbeat.

Challenge Yourself

Setting small, realistic, and positive goals can be a way to stay active and incrementally increase your fitness level. It is helpful to not only see what you have achieved, but also let you know when you are in a rut and need to reach out for motivation. Break your goals into small steps to climb the fitness ladder to success. If you have never exercised before and have been given the go-ahead by your doctor, a small goal of 5 or 10 minutes per day is an example of a great start. If you are already in the habit of exercising, set a goal of adding an additional 5 minutes to your session or adding an extra session into your week.

Hydrate and Fuel Your Workouts

Having the proper hydration and adequate fuel can make a big difference in your workout performance, but you don't need to overdo it either. Fuel and hydrate yourself appropriately before fitness to maximize your workout for blood sugar and weight control.

Water is your best bet for staying hydrated. A general guideline is to drink 2 cups within 2 hours of starting exercise and to drink at least ½ cup every 15 minutes during exercise. After more-intense workouts, drink 2–3 cups for every pound of fluid lost.

If you have worked up to doing more intense and longer-endurance exercise, then you may require some carbohydrates and electrolytes, and it would be a good idea to consult with a dietitian to create a plan. Don't run on empty; make sure you have eaten a snack or meal 1–2 hours before your workout. Ideally, eat something with a bit of carbohydrates and some protein, such as ½ banana, 1 rice cake with 1 tablespoon of peanut butter, or a light yogurt.

Now Is the Time

Don't delay in starting your fitness journey. Moving more is a critical step in improving insulin resistance and reducing any additional health risks. Put one foot in front of the other and make your body work its way to health! Check out the fitness resources in Appendix C for additional support.

CHAPTER 5

Other Lifestyle Adjustments and Your Plan for Beating Insulin Resistance

By now you know that maintaining a healthy weight, eating right, and exercising are important steps to managing your insulin resistance and improving your overall health. But there are also some other factors to consider when dealing with your diagnosis and formulating a successful treatment plan. Managing stress and mood, getting adequate rest and good-quality sleep, enjoying time with others for support, and developing good problem-solving skills all have a positive impact on your insulin resistance, weight, and overall health.

Being diagnosed with insulin resistance can have a significant emotional impact not just on you but on everyone who lives with and cares for you. Taking good care of yourself by recognizing stress and dealing with emotions and making time for enough rest, learning good coping techniques, and involving others in your journey will help you and those around you live a better, happier life. This chapter offers tips for how to address each aspect of emotional health.

Stress and Insulin Resistance

Experiencing stress doesn't feel good, and it can take a toll on both your mind and body. There are two types of stress: physical and mental. Physical stress occurs when significant demands are placed on the body, such as coping with illness, physical activity that is too intense, or recovering from surgery. Physical stress can have the potential to increase blood sugars and tax other body systems such as the heart. Mental stress originates in your mind—excessive worrying, for example. It also has the potential to wreak havoc on your body's systems, especially if it is chronic, repeated, and long-term.

When you face a physically or mentally stressful situation, your body starts a complex process of hormone release and reaction. The adrenal glands begin to pump out cortisol, the hormone primarily responsible for your physiological fight-or-flight reaction to situations you perceive as dangerous. Cortisol signals the liver to start up glucose production to give the brain and central nervous system added energy, while signaling the fat and muscle tissues to slow their uptake. At the same time, it causes the release of fatty acids from fat tissues, which are needed for muscle fuel, and sends your blood pressure up. Stress also prompts the adrenal glands to release epinephrine, the hormone that provides the adrenaline rush of the fight-or-flight reaction. High levels of circulating cortisol and epinephrine promote insulin resistance, in addition to ratcheting up blood sugar levels.

Since it increases blood pressure and glucose levels, stress is obviously no good for insulin resistance—or your health as a whole. In addition to impacting the body and blood sugars directly, stress can also be problematic indirectly because it may distract you from taking proper care of yourself. This is dangerous because it may take you off track from controlling your insulin resistance as you become preoccupied with other issues. It can also lead to unhealthy coping mechanisms such as overeating or drinking alcohol.

The Signs of Stress

Everyone reacts differently to stress. The following are some of the most common signs and symptoms that manifest as reactions to stress:

- **Physical:** fatigue, insomnia, muscle aches, heart palpitations, flushing/sweating, digestive disturbances/abdominal upset, headaches, increased or decreased appetite, frequent colds/illnesses, dry mouth
- **Mental:** anxiety/racing thoughts, difficulty concentrating, nervousness, memory loss, feeling worried/scared, feeling frustrated/short-tempered/irritable, feeling sad
- **Behavioral:** overeating, consuming alcohol, using drugs, becoming withdrawn, having emotional outbursts, pacing, developing nervous habits like nail-biting

Recognizing and becoming aware of when you are stressed and how your own stress manifests is one of the first steps in helping yourself. Consider which signs you may have experienced. Reflect on any that may be recurring, or if you tend to have more mental reactions to stress, or more physical or behavioral reactions.

Managing Stress

Studies have shown that stress-management programs can be extremely effective in not just improving psychological well-being, but also controlling blood sugar. One study published in *Diabetes Care* in 2002 found that just five sessions of stress-management training lowered HbA1c levels an average of half a percentage point. The study involved a stress-training regimen of audiotape-led progressive muscle relaxation, cognitive and behavioral therapy (including guided imagery and deep-breathing exercises), and education on the mechanisms and health consequences of stress.

In addition to guided relaxation, behavioral education, and therapy, there are many other techniques you can use to relieve stress. Using a combination of these tools—including the support of friends, family members, and professionals—is a crucial step in your journey to better health.

Harness the Power of Deep Breathing
If you find that you are feeling stressed, foggy, anxious, or upset, one of the best things you can do is to take a time-out to breathe. The simple act of just taking a few deep breaths can help calm your body and clear your mind, not to mention that it can do wonders for your blood sugar levels.

A simple breathing technique is to sit in a chair, close your eyes, and take a deep, slow breath through your nose. Hold it in for a few seconds and then breathe out fully and very slowly for a few seconds through your mouth. Repeat this up to five to ten times to help relax and reset.

Consider Meditation
It has been demonstrated that meditation can have positive effects on multiple areas in the body, including your metabolic, endocrine, and psychological systems. It can even lower insulin resistance, blood sugar, and hemoglobin A1c. Consider meditation to help clear your mind and relax your body for stress reduction. For guidance and instruction, try taking a meditation class. You can also use a meditation DVD, online tutorial, or app in the comfort of your own home.

Don't Go It Alone
If you are experiencing stress and worry, don't keep it inside and try to deal with it entirely by yourself. Turn to others in your support system in times of stress; it can make a big difference. Reach out for help by talking about your feelings with family, friends, or a colleague to vent and take advantage of companionship. Consider seeing a behavioral therapist for persistent stress and mood

changes such as depression or anxiety to discuss your issues and learn ways to cope. Think about joining a support group to interact with others who can identify with what you are going through. You might be surprised how relieved you feel after letting out what is bothering you, and it can certainly help you manage your insulin resistance as well.

Reframe Your Thoughts

If you find that negative or worrisome thoughts are bringing you down, try to replace them or put a positive spin on your thoughts instead. For example, if you are thinking, "I dread doing this project; it's so much work, and it's going to be terrible," instead try, "Wow, this project is going to be challenging, but I can do it. I will take it a step at a time, and it will feel awesome when I get it done." Sometimes it's helpful to have a mantra or upbeat saying that you can repeat to yourself over and over. Combining it with deep breathing can combat mental stress, which is key to blood sugar control.

Laugh and Smile More

Never underestimate the power of a good hearty laugh. Did you know that scientific studies have demonstrated the health benefits of laughter? These include helping cardiovascular functions and delaying complications in type 2 diabetes. It's true: Laughter causes positive changes that affect you for the better psychologically, biochemically, and in terms of your immunity. So, lighten up—your body and mind will thank you for it! Read a funny story, the comics, or watch a comedy show or movie. Tell jokes and funny stories around the table for some planned silliness with your family and friends.

Help Yourself by Helping Others

If you are feeling down, stressed, or in a rut, consider volunteering. Preliminary studies have shown that volunteering can lower depression and mortality and can increase feelings of well-being. Find a cause that you are interested in or passionate about such as helping animals, the elderly, or the less fortunate.

> **essential**
>
> Volunteering doesn't always have to be done through a formal organization; sometimes just taking time to help a family member, a friend, or a neighbor with a project or an errand can be a way of lending a hand.

Make sure you have a healthy life balance with volunteer work so it doesn't become too much for your schedule and actually cause stress. Decide on a regular time commitment that works best for you to help out.

Experiment with Other Coping Strategies

If you find yourself becoming stressed, know that it is not good for your insulin resistance—or your well-being. Besides trying some of the strategies discussed previously, such as meditation and laughing more, play around with other actions, including:

- Exercising
- Doing a hobby you enjoy, such as crafting or dancing
- Reading a good book
- Going out to see a movie
- Taking a warm bath
- Journaling your thoughts

See which activities may be the best fit for you and include them in your regular schedule. Any healthy habit you adopt to manage stress will also help you manage your insulin resistance.

Sleep and Insulin Resistance

The importance of a good night's sleep should never be underestimated. It can make all the difference to your physical and mental health. Adequate sleep quality and quantity are essential to maintaining several key processes in the body such as release of hormones, regulation of metabolism, control of appetite and weight, and upkeep of proper immune system and brain function. It is no wonder that sleep deprivation has been linked to a multitude of problems such as:

- Increased risk of diseases like cardiovascular disease, kidney disease, and obesity
- Susceptibility to infections, like the common cold

- Emotional and behavioral problems, like increased stress, reduced ability to learn and concentrate, and depression
- Lack of safety, such as more accidents and errors and issues with judgment

In addition, many studies have found that inadequate sleep is linked to metabolic changes that affect glucose levels and insulin resistance. These changes can lead to chronic problems such as type 2 diabetes. Specifically, inadequate sleep may affect levels of hormones that regulate appetite, leading to excessive food consumption, resulting in obesity.

question

How much sleep do I really need?

The amount of sleep your body requires varies with age. According to the National Sleep Foundation's expert panel, 7–8 hours of sleep is recommended for those 18 years and older.

It's not just the quantity of sleep you get that's important; the quality of your sleep also matters. The 2017 report by the National Sleep Foundation listed the key indicators of good-quality sleep as the following:

- Sleeping most of the time while in bed (at least 85 percent of total time)
- Falling asleep in 30 minutes or less
- Waking up no more than once per night

■ Being awake for 20 minutes or less after initially falling asleep

Consider whether your own sleeping patterns match up to these indicators of quality sleep.

Why Don't People Get Enough Sleep?

The modern lifestyle that is characterized by obsession with electronic devices, longer work hours, night-shift work, and longer waking hours of days packed with activities poses a huge challenge to getting adequate sleep.

> **fact**
>
> Obstructive sleep apnea (OSA) is a common sleep disorder that affects 3–7 percent of the population worldwide. Individuals with OSA experience blockages in the airway repeatedly during sleep, sometimes blocking breathing entirely. Common causes include a person's physical structure, such as large tonsils, or medical conditions like obesity. OSA may lead to impaired glucose tolerance and/or insulin sensitivity, so there is a higher prevalence of the condition among those with pre-diabetes and diabetes. OSA is most often treated by the use of breathing devices, as well as lifestyle changes.

According to a recent study in the Centers for Disease Control and Prevention's *Morbidity and Mortality Weekly Report*, more than a third of adult Americans are not getting adequate sleep on a regular basis. The reality is that for many, getting enough sleep is just not a priority. However, the potential for good rest is there if you take advantage of it.

For some, sleep disorders also create challenges to falling asleep and getting good-quality sleep. Common disorders that affect sleep include sleep apnea and insomnia. Even issues that may seem completely separate from sleep, such as generalized anxiety, heartburn, and thyroid disease, can make getting good-quality, adequate sleep a challenge.

Ensuring that you get enough sleep—and that it is good-quality sleep—will be an important step in your journey to better health and insulin resistance management.

Improving Sleep

If you are having trouble getting good-quality, adequate sleep, it is important to discuss it with your medical team so you can work together to try to find the causes and create a treatment plan. If you think you may have insomnia or other specific sleep problem, seeking help from a medical professional is especially crucial in treatment. Also be sure to explore the following helpful suggestions for promoting better sleep.

Create an Environment Conducive to Sleep

Check your room to determine if it is sleep-friendly. Do your best to create a comfortable bedroom that encourages sleep and helps you to promote control of your insulin resistance and health. Make sure your bed is large enough and your pillow is comfortable. A good mattress can be helpful and should not be older than 9 or 10 years.

Your room should be as dark and as quiet as possible. If it is not, then consider using a sleep blindfold, earplugs, or blackout curtains. You want to keep the room well ventilated and at the right temperature as well, not too hot or too cold for you.

Stick To a Regular Sleep Schedule

By keeping a habitual bedtime and waking time, you can help set your body's internal clock, referred to as a *circadian rhythm*, in your favor. This will help to get you adapted to a good sleep routine. Also, by keeping to a regular bedtime, your schedule can help ensure you will get to bed in time to get enough hours of sleep. Create a sleep schedule for more consistent rest as an important part of your lifestyle plan. Make every attempt to go to bed around the same time every night, even on the weekends, if possible. Try not to sleep in more than 1 or 2 hours maximum on the weekends or days off. Large shifts in your bedtime or waking hours can disrupt your circadian rhythm and cause problems with sleep, as well as your alertness and energy levels during the day.

If you are trying to adjust to an earlier bedtime, do it gradually in 15-minute intervals each night until the routine is comfortable. Have trouble waking up in the morning?

Let some morning sunlight in to help your internal body clock work with you to greet the day.

Develop a Calming Bedtime Ritual

Give yourself some time to wind down the hour before bed—your body and blood sugars will thank you for it. Avoid bright lights up to an hour before bedtime, and keep things as dim as possible to prevent disrupting your internal clock and to encourage sleepiness. Skip computers, TV, tablets, and cell phones up to an hour before turning in. The blue light they emit may be disruptive and keep you from falling asleep. Instead of using electronics, do some light reading, listen to music, talk with a loved one about your day, or even take a warm bath or shower to help relax your body and get ready for bed.

Exercise Regularly

By now you have learned about the benefits of exercise—it helps improve blood sugar control and weight. Well, it can also help you sleep! Specifically, it can help reduce stress, depression, and anxiety, and it may promote changes in body temperature, all of which can encourage sleep. Use regular exercise to promote body changes that promote sleep.

Avoid Sleep Saboteurs

Don't engage in behaviors that prevent sleep. These include:

1. **Caffeine.** Cut the coffee, tea, and cola before bed since they are stimulants. If

you must drink coffee, switch to decaf, but be aware it still has some caffeine. Watch foods and beverages containing chocolate as well, as it too has low levels of caffeine.

2. **Eating too little or too much food close to bedtime.** Being hungry before bed can make it difficult to turn in, but feeling stuffed can be uncomfortable and cause indigestion that may keep you awake.

3. **Late-afternoon naps.** Too much napping can disrupt your body's internal clock and make it difficult to get to sleep on time.

---

question

So when and how should I nap?

Napping the right way can help you re-energize without interfering with a good night's sleep. Keep naps short, no longer than 10-20 minutes, and try not to nap after 3 p.m.

Making the right choices for better sleep means making the right choices for your health.

Social Support and Insulin Resistance

Maintaining a social support network is good for your health and is another key component to helping you deal with your insulin resistance and manage it successfully. Countless studies have shown that having social support from others can have direct effects on health, such as helping with weight management and lowering stress and depression.

Social support can take on many forms, all of which can be beneficial in different ways. The types of social support that can help with managing insulin resistance specifically include:

- **Emotional support:** affection, love, care, empathy, trust-building
- **Esteem support:** encouragement of independence and reinforcement of self-care and skills and abilities
- **Informational support:** recommendations, advice, information
- **Tangible support:** help with tasks from others, financial assistance
- **Social network support:** sense of belonging to a group, companionship, and identification

Your support network can include family, friends, work colleagues, peers with your medical condition, and your healthcare team. (Check out Appendix C for online support group examples and suggestions.)

Nurturing Supportive Relationships

If you are lucky enough to have people around you offering love and support, embrace it and tell them how they can help. Use clear communication so your friends and family can get on the same page about what your needs are, and how they can best assist and support you. Be open and specific to eliminate any confusion or hesitation they may have as to how they can help. Give them examples of how to help. This can turn their good intentions into concrete actions that will benefit you and your relationship.

There are countless ways to nurture your bonds and encourage a healthy relationship that supports you and your needs—and allows you to support others in their needs too.

Make Time for Social Outings and Date Nights

With the busy lifestyles of the modern world, it is easy to get caught up in the monotony of your job(s) and other commitments, which can take too much time away from relationships with your partner, family, and friends. Carving out regular time is important to maintaining love and social connections that strengthen bonds and maintain the support network that is so beneficial to your mental and physical health. Taking this time can help you succeed in managing your insulin resistance.

Schedule outings with your family so you can spend quality time together to talk, laugh, and enjoy each other's company. Plan a regular date night with your partner to take time out to connect and have fun without distractions. Spend a day with friends, catching up and reminiscing.

Consider Counseling

If constant clashes are creating tension and stress between you and your partner or with other members of your family, then consider going to counseling together. Get some guidance on how to create stronger and healthier relationships; stress can take a toll on your blood sugar, weight, and health, so getting to the root of your problems and working things out sooner than later will benefit your health, as well as those around you. Look for a therapist who specializes in marriage and family therapy.

Learn about Treatment Together

The diagnosis of insulin resistance can be overwhelming and emotional. Let your partner, family, and friends take the journey with you by learning more about the condition and the lifestyle changes that are required. Having your partner and/or family members at medical appointments can be helpful. It's good to have more than one set of ears in case you have trouble remembering or understanding recommendations. If you and your friends and family are all clear on the condition and its treatment plan, you'll be more effective in managing your insulin resistance.

Let others go with you to your appointment with the dietitian, especially if your partner does the cooking or the grocery shopping. That way they can support your meal plan. Remind yourself that it can be a positive experience to have others on your team as you are starting to get familiar with insulin resistance and how to tackle it.

Use Online Resources

There is a wealth of information on just about any subject on the Internet. This is also the case for insulin resistance, pre-diabetes, and diabetes. Using online information and support can be helpful as resources to enhance your lifestyle treatment plan. If you have a question, get in the habit of looking up the answer. Take advantage of the Internet to get more information about your condition and for helpful lifestyle change ideas—especially recipes and menu ideas. As long as you take what you read with a grain of salt, you certainly stand more to gain than you can lose.

There are also many online groups for people with insulin resistance, pre-diabetes, diabetes, and obesity, and they can be almost as—if not more—supportive and informative than real-time groups. There's input from Pennsylvania to Paris, with participants from all walks of life and a broad range of experience with these health conditions. And the beauty of an online support group is that it is there all day and all night for your questions, vents, and gripes.

Make Lifestyle Change a Family Affair

Everyone in the household can benefit from eating a healthy diet, getting more activity, getting more sleep, and engaging in positive behavior for health. The family that sticks to important lifestyle changes stays healthy together! Get everyone on board with your plan so there is less temptation to eat the wrong things or slack off on activity. Do healthy activities together like going shopping and cooking a nutritious meal, doing group exercise sessions like biking or hiking, and taking time out to relax as a family with upbeat activities like a game night or a dance party.

A 10-Week Plan for Reversing Insulin Resistance

Now that you have explored key influences on insulin resistance such as diet, activity, and weight loss, it is time to take action. The following 10-week plan to kick insulin resistance is designed to help you set modest goals and put what you have learned into practice. Each week includes a healthy lifestyle theme along with suggested goals to help you achieve success.

Week 1: Check Your Portions

Portion control is everything, even when you choose healthy foods! If you eat large portions, you will have trouble controlling your calories. Using the plate method (see Chapter 3) at lunch and dinner, fill half of your plate with vegetables, one-quarter of the plate with starches, and one-quarter of the plate with meat or meat substitute. A serving of milk and fruit should also be added to each meal.

Your Goals for Week 1
- Give the plate method a try to reduce portion sizes
- For several days, measure or weigh your food to see just how much you are eating

Week 2: Eat More Vegetables and Fruit Every Day

The DASH recommendation to eat 4–5 servings each of fruit and vegetables every day sounds like a lot of food, but once you know how to incorporate these foods into your plan it becomes easy. Why that many servings? Because fruit and vegetables are nutrient-dense foods with high fiber and lower calories.

Your Goals for Week 2
- Take two pieces of fruit from home each day to have for a midday snack or with lunch
- Keep raw vegetables washed, cut up, and ready to eat for quick snacks or salads

Week 3: Get Walking

Start walking, even if you are only able to manage a few minutes at a time. Aim to walk most days of the week, and make sure that you have comfortable walking shoes or sneakers.

Your Goals for Week 3
- Walk for as long as you are comfortably able to
- Keep a written record of when and how long you are walking
- Wear a pedometer so you can track how many steps you take, and use that number as a motivator to help you increase it each day

Week 4: Switch to Whole Grains

Begin to switch out the white flour and white grain products in your kitchen for whole-grain foods. Whole grains provide more fiber and nutrients and have less impact on your blood glucose. Look for products that list whole-grain flour rather than enriched flour as one of the first ingredients.

Your Goals for Week 4
- Add whole-grain pasta or brown rice to a favorite dish or in combination with vegetables or beans
- Purchase a new whole-grain food that you haven't used (e.g., quinoa, kasha, or bulgur) before and try it as a replacement for rice, pasta, or potatoes

Week 5: Manage Your Stress

Take stress seriously and find ways to reduce it. Chronic stress can wreak havoc on health and well-being by lowering your immunity and making you more susceptible to many types of illness.

Your Goals for Week 5

- Add stretching exercises, meditation, or deep breathing exercises to your daily routine
- Allow yourself some downtime from the daily grind each day and spend that time enjoying a relaxing activity

Week 6: Get Adequate Sleep

Insufficient sleep can have a negative impact on your health. In fact, poor-quality sleep on a regular basis can contribute to insulin resistance, metabolic syndrome, and diabetes—just what you are trying to avoid!

Your Goals for Week 6

- Make enough time to get 7–8 hours of sleep each night
- Develop good sleeping habits by rising and retiring about the same time each day, and avoid distractions such as TV at times when you should be going to sleep

Week 7: Don't Forget the Snacks

Having meals and snacks at regular times can go a long way toward controlling your appetite and blood glucose. Snacking during the day is fine, as long as you make good choices that are low in calories and have nutritional value.

Your Goals for Week 7

- Buy healthy snacks to have on hand at all times
- If necessary, prepare snacks ahead of time so they are always ready to go (cut up vegetables, premeasure nuts into individual containers, etc.)

Week 8: Ramp Up Your Exercise

You may have started an exercise plan already, but it's time to take it up a notch. This is important because exercising the same muscles or at the same intensity all the time will eventually stall your efforts at weight loss.

Your Goals for Week 8

- Turn your moderate walk into a brisk walk and add additional steps
- Add weight bearing exercises to your routine in addition to walking, such as squats or wall push-ups

Week 9: Change Your Food Behaviors

Negative food habits are not always easy to change. Make a conscious effort to correct eating habits that cause you to get off track.

Your Goals for Week 9

- Slow down when you eat and take the time to enjoy every bite
- Drink plenty of water

Week 10: Put It All Together

Monitor your overall progress by looking at how well you have done with various aspects of your plan.

Your Goals for Week 10
- Make a list of all the things you have been able to achieve, as well as the goals that still need work: Seeing in writing all that you have accomplished is very satisfying and motivates you to keep going
- Congratulate and reward yourself for a job well done!

Next Steps

The coming chapters provide you with a plethora of healthy recipes to help you succeed. To continue the work you have done over these past 10 weeks, also consider using the meal plan at the back of this book (Appendix A) to keep you focused on healthy food choices. And when you need to find encouragement to stay the course, join one of the online support groups mentioned in Appendix C. Share your love of healthy eating by bringing one of the recipes to your next potluck or holiday gathering!

Also keep in mind that while health is at the forefront of the following recipes, we have aimed to create dishes that anyone, anywhere can make and enjoy. Even though we provide specific ingredients and equipment, most of the time, what you have on hand is a perfectly acceptable substitute. So don't worry about the type of potato or tomato; just give it a try!

CHAPTER 6

Breakfast and Brunch

Bacon and Egg Breakfast Fried Rice

This special breakfast is easy to make, and it reheats well for leftovers, so go ahead and double or triple the batch! It has a good amount of protein, includes a whole grain, and is low in fat. You can add a dash of salt and pepper and low-fat cheese if you like.

SERVES 4

Per Serving:

Calories	100
Fat	5g
Saturated Fat	2g
Sodium	250mg
Carbohydrates	7g
Fiber	1g
Sugar	0g
Protein	5g

1 teaspoon salted butter, divided
½ cup chopped cooked turkey bacon
⅓ cup diced scallions
1 large egg, beaten
1½ cups cooked brown rice

1 Melt ½ teaspoon butter in a large skillet or wok over medium-high heat. Add bacon and scallions and sauté 3–5 minutes until slightly browned. Remove bacon mixture from pan and set aside.

2 Melt remaining ½ teaspoon butter in same skillet over medium heat. Add egg to pan and cook, stirring, until set, about 2 minutes.

3 Stir in reserved bacon mixture and rice. Sauté 3–4 minutes until rice is lightly browned. Serve immediately.

Great Greek Omelet

Liven up egg whites with the Mediterranean flavors of oregano, sun-dried tomatoes, and olives. Serve with fresh fruit for breakfast or with a side of mixed greens for a light, protein-packed lunch.

½ cup liquid egg whites

½ cup chopped fresh spinach

½ teaspoon dried oregano

1 tablespoon chopped sun-dried tomatoes

5 kalamata olives, pitted and chopped

¼ cup shredded low-fat mozzarella cheese

1 Spray a medium skillet with nonstick cooking spray and heat over medium heat 1 minute.

2 Pour in egg whites and cook over medium heat 1 minute. Top one side of egg whites with spinach, oregano, tomatoes, olives, and cheese and cook 1 minute more.

3 Fold omelet to cover toppings and cook 1 minute, flip over and cook about 1 minute more until lightly browned. Serve immediately.

SERVES 1	
Per Serving:	
Calories	230
Fat	12g
Saturated Fat	3.5g
Sodium	790mg
Carbohydrates	11g
Fiber	1g
Sugar	2g
Protein	21g

SUBSTITUTING WHOLE EGGS FOR EGG WHITES

You can replace the egg whites in this recipe with two whole eggs, but keep in mind that the amounts of calories, fat, and cholesterol will be increased substantially.

Super Greens Crustless Quiche

This delicious quiche provides a full serving of vegetables for breakfast. Leftovers will keep in the refrigerator for up to 3 days for a quick breakfast or lunch whenever you choose.

1 tablespoon olive oil

½ large white onion, peeled and thinly sliced

1 cup chopped kale

1 cup chopped Swiss chard

1 cup chopped beet greens, cut into thin strips

1 clove garlic, peeled and minced

4 large eggs

4 large egg whites

¼ cup shredded Italian cheese blend

1 Preheat oven to 350°F. Spray a 9" pie pan with nonstick cooking spray.

2 Heat oil in a large skillet over medium heat 30 seconds. Add onion and sauté until soft, about 5 minutes.

3 Add kale, Swiss chard, and beet greens to skillet and sauté 2 minutes until wilted. Add garlic and cook, stirring often, until greens are softened, another 3 minutes. Remove from heat and set aside.

4 In a large bowl, beat together eggs and egg whites. Stir in cheese and cooked greens.

5 Pour mixture into prepared pie pan and bake 30 minutes or until quiche is brown around the edges.

6 Cool quiche in pan on a wire rack for 3 minutes before slicing and serving.

Buckwheat Pancakes

These classic low-fat pancakes are bursting with the hearty flavor of whole grains. Top them with your favorite chopped fruit and a dollop of Greek yogurt for a real treat.

1 cup whole-wheat flour

½ cup buckwheat flour

1½ teaspoons baking powder

2 large egg whites

¼ cup apple juice concentrate

1½ cups skim milk, divided

1 Sift flours and baking powder together in a large bowl. Combine egg whites, apple juice concentrate, and 1¼ cups milk in a separate medium bowl.

2 Add milk mixture to dry ingredients; mix well, but do not overmix. Add remaining milk if necessary to reach desired consistency.

3 Preheat a large nonstick skillet or griddle greased with nonstick cooking spray over medium heat for 1 minute. Pour in batter in pancake shapes and cook 1–2 minutes on each side until lightly browned.

SERVES 4	
Per Serving:	
Calories	230
Fat	1.5g
Saturated Fat	0g
Sodium	75mg
Carbohydrates	44g
Fiber	5g
Sugar	15g
Protein	11g

NOT YOUR AVERAGE GRAIN

Buckwheat is part of the same family as quinoa and amaranth, and though it has "wheat" in its name it does not contain wheat at all. It adds a nice earthy flavor to recipes.

Tomato and Basil Baked Egg Cups

SERVES 12

Per Serving:

Calories	50
Fat	3g
Saturated Fat	1g
Sodium	75mg
Carbohydrates	1g
Fiber	0g
Sugar	0g
Protein	5g

These egg cups are surprisingly easy to make and taste great with a dash of salt and pepper. Keep them in the refrigerator for up to 1 week and reheat them in the microwave for a quick, fuss-free breakfast, lunch, or dinner.

6 large eggs

½ cup liquid egg whites

3 tablespoons grated Parmesan cheese

1 cup halved cherry tomatoes

¼ cup chopped fresh basil

1 Preheat oven to 350°F. Spray a twelve-cup muffin tin with non-stick cooking spray.

2 In a large bowl, whisk eggs, egg whites, and cheese until light and fluffy. Stir in tomatoes and basil.

3 Pour mixture into cups of prepared muffin tin and bake 22 minutes or until eggs are set, firm, and lightly browned. Serve warm or at room temperature.

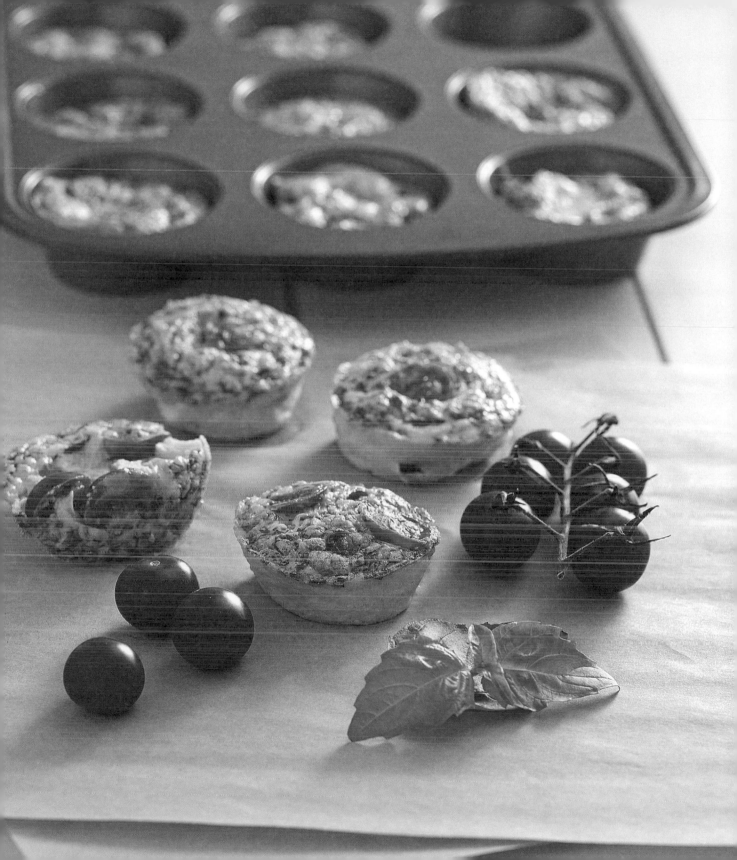

Egg White Pancakes

SERVES 2

Per Serving:

Calories	150
Fat	1.5g
Saturated Fat	0g
Sodium	110mg
Carbohydrates	23g
Fiber	2g
Sugar	6g
Protein	10g

CREATIVE TOPPINGS

Experiment with toast and pancake toppings. Try a tablespoon of raisins, almonds, apples, bananas, berries, peanuts, pears, walnuts, or wheat germ. Or add a teaspoon of your favorite nut butter.

All you need are a few simple wholesome ingredients to create these delicious high-protein pancakes. You won't be able to tell they are healthy.

4 large egg whites
½ cup rolled oats
4 teaspoons reduced-calorie or low-sugar strawberry jam
1 teaspoon confectioners' sugar

1 Put all ingredients except confectioners' sugar in a blender and process until smooth.
2 Spray a large nonstick skillet with nonstick cooking spray and heat over medium heat 30 seconds. Pour half of mixture into pan; cook 4 minutes.
3 Flip pancake and cook until the inside is cooked, about 2 minutes. Transfer to a large plate and repeat with remaining batter. Dust each pancake with confectioners' sugar before serving.

Vegetable Frittata

This frittata is a great way to add protein and vegetables to your morning. Or add a side of mixed greens for an easy and delicious lunch option.

1½ tablespoons olive oil

½ cup chopped red bell pepper

3 large eggs

4 ounces egg substitute (or egg whites)

4 ounces asparagus, woody ends trimmed, cut diagonally in 1" pieces

¾ cup cooked cubed Russet potatoes, peels on

⅓ cup crumbled feta cheese

1 teaspoon dried oregano

SERVES 4	
Per Serving:	
Calories	180
Fat	11g
Saturated Fat	4g
Sodium	220mg
Carbohydrates	9g
Fiber	1g
Sugar	2g
Protein	11g

1 Preheat oven to 350°F.

2 Heat oil in a large ovenproof nonstick skillet over medium heat 30 seconds. Add bell pepper and cook until softened, about 3 minutes.

3 In a medium bowl, beat together eggs and egg substitute. Add asparagus, potatoes, cheese, and oregano.

4 Pour egg mixture into skillet and stir until eggs on the bottom of pan begin to set, about 3 minutes. Gently pull cooked eggs from side of skillet, allowing uncooked egg on top to come in contact with heated skillet. Repeat, working all around skillet, until most of eggs on top have begun to set, about 8 minutes.

5 Transfer skillet to oven and bake until top is set and dry to the touch, about 4 minutes. Loosen frittata around edges of skillet and transfer onto a serving plate.

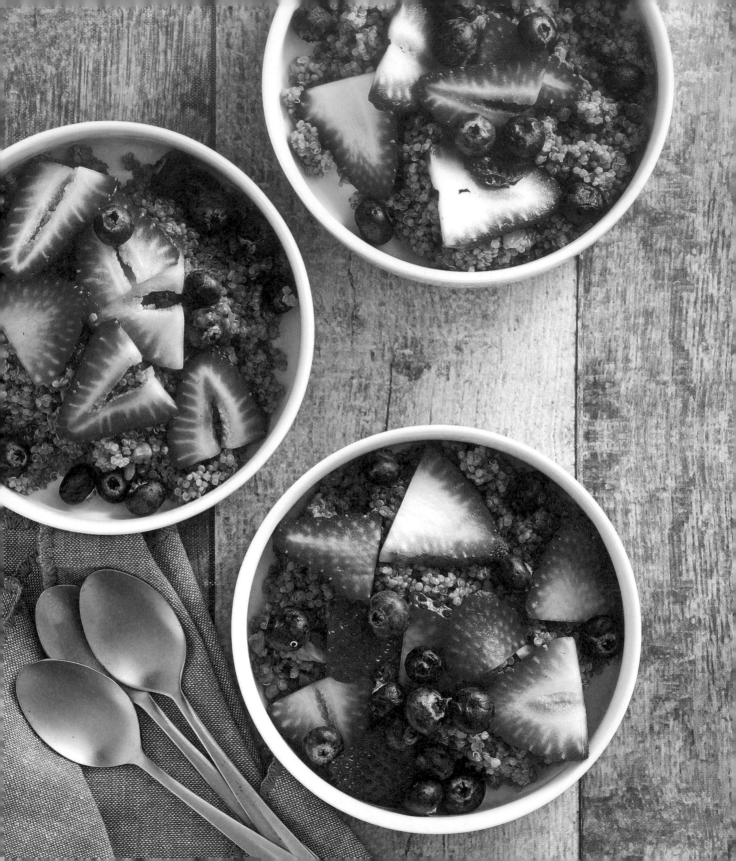

Quinoa Berry Breakfast

Try other berries, nuts, or spices such as ginger or nutmeg to vary this nutritious breakfast cereal. Top it with a healthy plant-based milk for a filling and delicious alternative to oatmeal.

1 cup quinoa, rinsed

2 cups water

¼ cup chopped walnuts

1 teaspoon ground cinnamon

1 cup fresh blueberries

1 cup hulled and sliced fresh strawberries

1　Place quinoa, water, walnuts, and cinnamon in a 1½-quart sauce-pan and bring to a boil over high heat. Once boiling, reduce heat to low, cover, and cook 15 minutes or until all water has been absorbed.

2　Serve topped with berries.

SERVES 4	
Per Serving:	
Calories	240
Fat	8g
Saturated Fat	1g
Sodium	10mg
Carbohydrates	37g
Fiber	5g
Sugar	7g
Protein	8g

SINGLE-SERVING QUICK TIP

Use this basic recipe to make four servings at once. Refrigerate any leftover portions; micro-wave 1–1½ minutes on high for single portions as needed. Use cooked quinoa within 3 days.

Whole-Wheat Zucchini Bread

SERVES 20

Per Serving:

Calories	140
Fat	6g
Saturated Fat	0.5g
Sodium	190mg
Carbohydrates	21g
Fiber	2g
Sugar	8g
Protein	3g

For a little twist on this recipe, ⅓ cup dried cranberries, currants, raisins, or chopped nuts can be added in place of the sunflower seeds.

2 large eggs

2 tablespoons liquid egg whites

½ cup amber honey

2 cups shredded zucchini

⅔ cup unsweetened applesauce

⅓ cup canola oil

2 teaspoons vanilla extract

2 cups whole-wheat pastry flour

1 cup all-purpose flour

¼ cup Splenda (granulated)

1 teaspoon salt

2 teaspoons baking powder

1 teaspoon baking soda

2 teaspoons ground cinnamon

½ teaspoon ground nutmeg

⅓ cup sunflower seeds, toasted

1 Preheat oven to 350°F. Spray four mini loaf pans with nonstick cooking spray.

2 In a large mixing bowl, beat eggs and egg whites until foamy. Mix in honey, zucchini, applesauce, oil, and vanilla.

3 In a separate large mixing bowl, sift together pastry flour, all-purpose flour, Splenda, salt, baking powder, baking soda, cinnamon, and nutmeg.

4 Gradually add dry ingredients to zucchini mixture; mix until all ingredients are combined, but do not overmix. Stir in sunflower seeds.

5 Divide batter evenly into prepared pans. Bake 35 minutes or until tops are browned and a toothpick inserted in the center comes out clean.

6 Cool bread in pans on a wire rack 10 minutes. Turn loaves out onto rack and cool completely, about 30 minutes, before slicing. Store in an airtight container in the refrigerator up to 5 days.

Mini Orange Date Loaves

These lovely little loaves make a nice treat for breakfast or an afternoon snack. They also make a healthy gift to pass along to friends during the holidays—just wrap them up in parchment paper and tie them with colorful string or ribbon.

2 tablespoons frozen orange juice concentrate

2 tablespoons grated orange zest

¾ cup chopped dates

½ cup light brown sugar

¼ cup granulated sugar

1 cup nonfat plain yogurt

1 large egg

1¼ cups all-purpose flour

¾ cup whole-wheat flour

1 teaspoon baking soda

1 teaspoon baking powder

½ teaspoon salt

1 tablespoon vegetable oil

1 teaspoon vanilla extract

1   Preheat oven to 350°F. Spray four mini loaf pans with nonstick cooking spray.

2   In a food processor, pulse orange juice concentrate, orange zest, dates, sugars, yogurt, and egg until mixed. Add remaining ingredients; pulse until mixed, scraping down sides of bowl if necessary.

3   Divide mixture among prepared pans; spread mixture so each pan has an even layer. Bake 15 minutes or until a toothpick inserted in the center comes out clean.

4   Cool bread in pans on a wire rack 10 minutes. Turn loaves out onto rack and cool to room temperature, about 30 minutes, before serving. Store covered in the refrigerator up to 1 week.

SERVES 20

Per Serving:

Calories	110
Fat	1g
Saturated Fat	0g
Sodium	125mg
Carbohydrates	23g
Fiber	1g
Sugar	12g
Protein	2g

ARE YOUR EYES BIGGER THAN YOUR STOMACH?

When you use mini loaf pans, it's much easier to arrive at the recommended serving size while still enjoying a full slice. There's a psychological advantage to getting a full rather than half slice!

Carrot Zucchini Spice Muffins

With both fruit and vegetables, these muffins are a perfect balance of sweet and savory. Enjoy with tea as an afternoon snack, or freeze and reheat for a warm breakfast any day.

2 cups old-fashioned rolled oats

¾ cup all-purpose flour

1 teaspoon baking powder

½ teaspoon baking soda

2 teaspoons ground cinnamon

3 large overripe bananas, peeled and mashed

6 tablespoons liquid egg whites

6 tablespoons packed light brown sugar

¼ cup skim milk

1 tablespoon vanilla extract

½ cup finely grated carrot

½ cup finely grated zucchini

½ cup finely grated red apple

1 Preheat oven to 350°F. Spray a twelve-cup muffin tin with non-stick cooking spray.

2 Combine oats, flour, baking powder, baking soda, and cinnamon in a small bowl.

3 In a large bowl, beat together mashed banana, egg whites, sugar, milk, and vanilla. Stir in carrot, zucchini, and apple.

4 Gradually add oat mixture to carrot mixture just enough to combine ingredients. Do not overmix. Spoon into prepared muffin tin.

5 Bake on bottom rack of oven 30 minutes or until muffin tops are lightly browned and firm and a toothpick inserted in the center comes out clean.

6 Cool in muffin tin at least 10 minutes before removing from tin. Store in an airtight container in the refrigerator for up to 3 days.

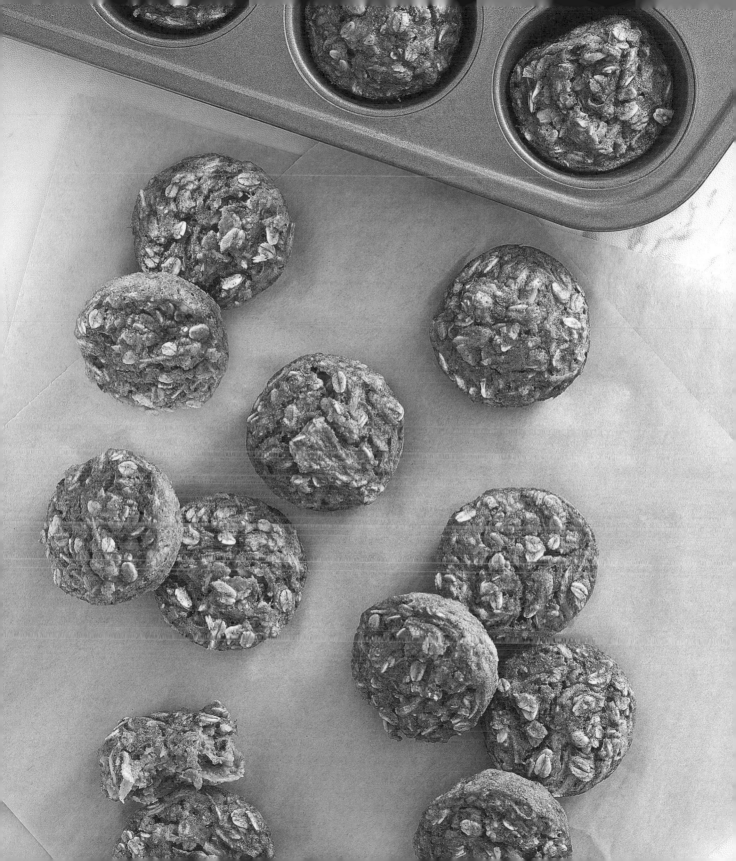

Banana Walnut Protein Muffins

SERVES 6

Per Serving:

Calories	420
Fat	8g
Saturated Fat	1g
Sodium	110mg
Carbohydrates	59g
Fiber	7g
Sugar	17g
Protein	23g

These moist large muffins are best eaten on the day you bake them, but leftovers can be stored in the refrigerator for up to 3 days. Reheat them in the microwave 30–40 seconds for a warm treat anytime.

2 cups old-fashioned rolled oats

¾ cup oat flour

¾ teaspoon baking powder

¼ teaspoon baking soda

6 tablespoons unflavored protein powder

3 large overripe bananas, peeled and mashed

6 tablespoons liquid egg whites

¼ cup packed light brown sugar

¼ cup skim milk

1 tablespoon vanilla extract

⅓ cup finely chopped walnuts

1 Preheat oven to 350°F. Spray a muffin tin with six large cups (or six small ovenproof ramekins) with nonstick cooking spray.

2 Combine oats, oat flour, baking powder, baking soda, and protein powder in a medium bowl.

3 In a large bowl, mix together mashed banana, egg whites, sugar, milk, and vanilla.

4 Add oat mixture to banana mixture and mix well. Fold in walnuts. Spoon batter into prepared muffin cups.

5 Bake on bottom rack of oven 30 minutes or until muffin tops are lightly browned and a toothpick inserted in the center comes out clean.

6 Cool muffins in pan on a wire rack 5 minutes, then remove them from pan. Serve warm or at room temperature.

CHAPTER 7

Appetizers and Snacks

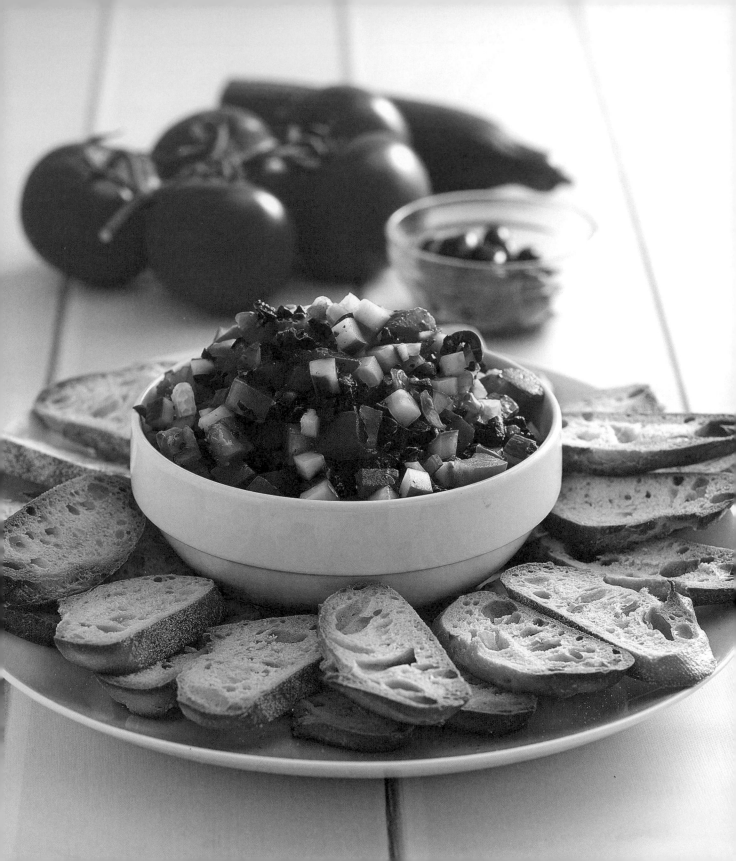

Mediterranean Bruschetta Mix

This recipe combines a few simple ingredients to create a delicious, low-calorie appetizer. Serve it with thinly sliced toasted bread, crackers, or pita bread. Add a dash of salt and pepper and some chopped oregano to kick up the flavor.

1 cup diced cucumber

1 cup diced Roma tomatoes

1 cup diced black olives

1 tablespoon rice vinegar

1 tablespoon lemon juice

Combine all ingredients in a medium bowl. Serve immediately or refrigerate covered up to 3 days.

SERVES 6	
Per Serving:	
Calories	45
Fat	3.5g
Saturated Fat	0g
Sodium	210mg
Carbohydrates	4g
Fiber	0g
Sugar	2g
Protein	0g

Spicy Almond Dip

MAKES ½ CUP

Per Serving (2 tablespoons):

Calories	70
Fat	5g
Saturated Fat	0g
Sodium	70mg
Carbohydrates	5g
Fiber	1g
Sugar	2g
Protein	2g

ADD MORE CRUNCH

Top this dip with chopped almonds to change up the texture and add some flair for serving.

Serve this unique dip with a kick as a healthy appetizer at parties or to liven up your favorite raw vegetables for a special snack.

¼ cup ground raw almonds

2 teaspoons Worcestershire sauce

½ teaspoon amber honey

½ teaspoon chili powder

1 teaspoon poppy seeds

½ teaspoon onion powder

2 tablespoons water

⅛ teaspoon ground black pepper

Place all ingredients in a food processor and blend until smooth. Serve at room temperature or refrigerate covered at least 2 hours before serving. Store any extra dip in an airtight container in the refrigerator for up to 3 days.

Italian-Style Bean Dip

Use this dip as an alternative to classic hummus. It's great for dipping, atop salads, or spread on sandwiches and wraps.

3 cups cooked white beans

½ teaspoon ground cumin

1 tablespoon lemon juice

1 tablespoon dried parsley

¼ teaspoon dried basil

1 teaspoon onion powder

¼ teaspoon garlic powder

1 tablespoon amber honey

Combine all ingredients in a food processor or blender and process until smooth. Add 1 teaspoon water if needed to thin dip. Serve or refrigerate in an airtight container up to 3 days.

MAKES 2 CUPS	
Per Serving (2 tablespoons):	
Calories	45
Fat	0g
Saturated Fat	0g
Sodium	0mg
Carbohydrates	8g
Fiber	2g
Sugar	1g
Protein	3g

Mushroom Caviar

MAKES 3 CUPS

Per Serving (2
tablespoons):

Calories	20
Fat	1.5g
Saturated Fat	0g
Sodium	120mg
Carbohydrates	1g
Fiber	0g
Sugar	0g
Protein	1g

DRY-ROASTED GARLIC

To dry-roast a head of
garlic: Preheat oven to
350°F and lightly spray
a small covered bak-
ing dish with nonstick
cooking spray. Slice off
½" from the top of the
garlic head. Rub off
any loose skin, being
careful not to separate
the cloves. Place in the
baking dish, cut-side up.
(If roasting more than 1
head, arrange them in
the dish so they don't
touch.) Cover and bake
until the garlic cloves
are tender when pierced,
about 30–40 minutes.
Roasted garlic heads will
keep in the refrigerator
for up to 3 days.

Serve this warm and savory dip with toasted bread. It can be made ahead of time and refrigerated for up to 3 days.

1½ cups chopped portobello mushrooms
1½ cups chopped white button mushrooms
¼ cup chopped scallions
4 cloves dry-roasted garlic, peeled
1 teaspoon lemon juice
½ teaspoon balsamic vinegar
1 tablespoon extra-virgin olive oil
½ teaspoon chopped fresh thyme
½ teaspoon sea salt
½ teaspoon ground black pepper

1 Place mushrooms and scallions in a medium microwave-safe bowl, cover, and microwave on high 1 minute. Rotate bowl and microwave in 30-second intervals until tender.
2 Transfer mushrooms and scallions to a food processor. (Reserve any liquid to use for thinning, if necessary.) Pulse several times to chop mixture, scraping down sides of bowl as needed. Add remaining ingredients and pulse until mixed.
3 Serve warm.

Snack Mix

This mix is infinitely variable. Use your favorite unsweetened cereals, swap the peanuts for almonds or walnuts, or add a salt-free seasoning blend to make it your own.

2 cups Wheat Chex cereal

2 cups Rice Chex cereal

2 cups Corn Chex cereal

1 cup mini pretzels

⅔ cup dry-roasted peanuts

2 tablespoons salted butter, melted

2 tablespoons olive oil

1 tablespoon Worcestershire sauce

¼ teaspoon garlic powder

⅛ teaspoon Tabasco sauce

1 Preheat oven to 300°F.

2 In a large bowl, combine cereals, pretzels, and peanuts.

3 In a separate medium bowl, combine butter, oil, Worcestershire sauce, garlic powder, and Tabasco sauce. Pour over cereal mixture; toss to coat evenly.

4 Spread mixture on a large ungreased baking sheet and bake 30 minutes, stirring every 10 minutes, until crisp and dry.

5 Cool about 40 minutes on baking sheet, then store in an airtight container at room temperature up to 3 days.

SERVES 16	
Per Serving:	
Calories	130
Fat	7g
Saturated Fat	1.5g
Sodium	170mg
Carbohydrates	16g
Fiber	1g
Sugar	2g
Protein	3g

Zesty Black Bean Salsa

SERVES 10

Per Serving:

Calories	80
Fat	3g
Saturated Fat	0g
Sodium	5mg
Carbohydrates	11g
Fiber	4g
Sugar	3g
Protein	3g

BEANS IN PLACE OF BEANS

All out of black beans? Just about any type of beans would work well in this salsa. Try pinto beans, small white beans, or even chickpeas.

Black beans add a hearty texture and tons of fiber to this fresh-tasting salsa. It makes a great accompaniment to chicken or shrimp.

1 cup chopped red onion

¼ cup chopped fresh cilantro

¼ cup chopped fresh parsley

3 tablespoons minced jalapeño pepper

1½ cups cooked black beans

4 cups chopped Roma tomatoes

3 tablespoons lime juice

2 tablespoons olive oil

1 Place onion, cilantro, parsley, and jalapeño in a food processor; chop finely.

2 In a medium bowl, combine onion mixture, black beans, and tomatoes.

3 In a separate small bowl, whisk together lime juice and oil. Pour over salsa and mix well.

4 Refrigerate covered at least 2 hours before serving, or store in an airtight container in the refrigerator up to 2 days.

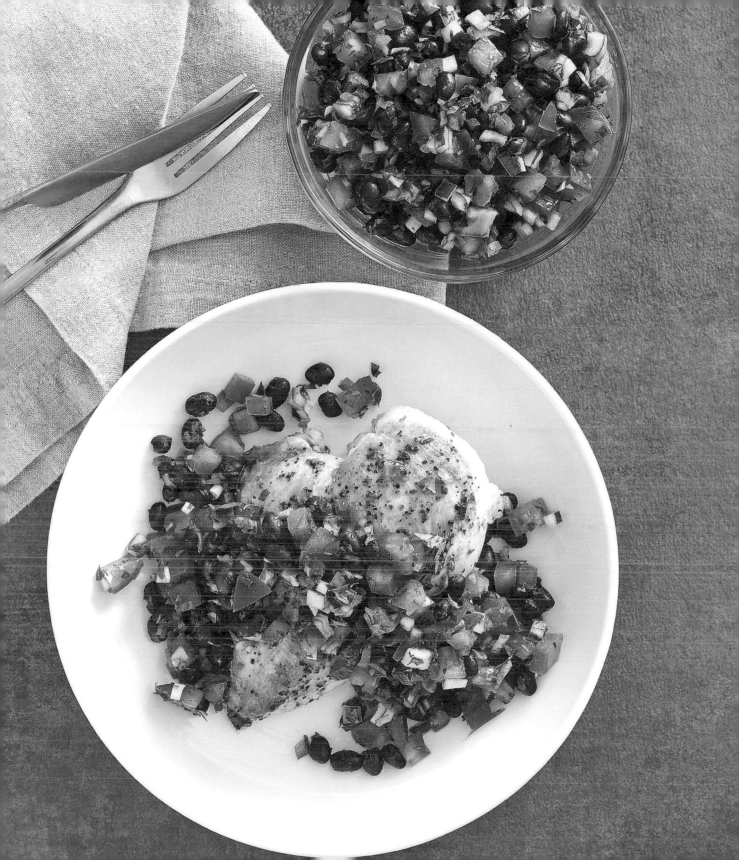

Asian Popcorn

SERVES 1	
Per Serving:	
Calories	140
Fat	2g
Saturated Fat	0g
Sodium	200mg
Carbohydrates	29g
Fiber	5g
Sugar	1g
Protein	5g

Because there are no oils, air-popped popcorn will keep for weeks if you store it in an airtight container. Pop a large batch and keep some on hand for later. Add in your favorite flavors for a warm, healthy snack anytime.

4 cups air-popped popcorn

Butter-flavored cooking spray

1 teaspoon low-sodium soy sauce

2 teaspoons lemon juice

1 teaspoon Chinese five-spice powder

¼ teaspoon ground coriander

¼ teaspoon garlic powder

1 Preheat oven to 250°F. Spread popcorn on a large nonstick baking sheet; lightly coat popcorn with cooking spray.

2 Mix together soy sauce, lemon juice, five-spice powder, coriander, and garlic powder in a small bowl. Drizzle over popcorn; lightly toss to coat evenly.

3 Bake 5 minutes, then toss popcorn, rotate pan, and bake an additional 5 minutes. Serve warm.

Deviled Eggs with Capers

A protein-packed appetizer or snack, these deviled eggs have the added flavor of capers as a delicious twist.

6 large hard-cooked eggs, peeled and cut in half lengthwise

½ cup light mayonnaise

1 teaspoon Tabasco sauce

1 teaspoon celery salt

1 teaspoon onion powder

1 teaspoon garlic powder

1 small chili pepper, seeded and finely minced

2 tablespoons extra-small capers

1 tablespoon chopped fresh chives

1 Scoop out egg yolks and place them in a food processor along with mayonnaise, Tabasco sauce, celery salt, onion powder, garlic powder, chili pepper, and capers. Blend until smooth.

2 Place egg whites on a large plate and spoon egg-yolk mixture into the hollows. Sprinkle eggs with chives. Cover with foil, tented above the egg-yolk mixture, and refrigerate at least 3 hours before serving, or store covered in the refrigerator for up to 3 days.

SERVES 12	
Per Serving:	
Calories	60
Fat	4g
Saturated Fat	1g
Sodium	260mg
Carbohydrates	2g
Fiber	0g
Sugar	1g
Protein	3g

BRINE-PACKED CAPERS

Capers are actually berries that have been pickled. You can get them packed in salt, or packed in brine. You can get larger ones or very small ones; the tiny ones have more flavor.

Quinoa-Stuffed Mushrooms

SERVES 12

Per Serving:

Calories	40
Fat	2g
Saturated Fat	1g
Sodium	80mg
Carbohydrates	3g
Fiber	0g
Sugar	1g
Protein	2g

LIGHTENING UP AN OLD FAVORITE

Most traditional stuffed-mushroom recipes call for less-than-healthy ingredients like refined white bread crumbs and full-fat cream cheese, as well as pork sausage and bacon. This version, stuffed with quinoa, low-fat cream cheese, turkey bacon, and just a touch of Parmesan cheese, is low in fat and calories, but high in flavor!

For a bit of a twist, substitute darker cremini mushrooms for the button mushrooms to bring an earthier flavor to this recipe.

1 teaspoon olive oil

3 tablespoons finely chopped white onion

2 slices turkey bacon, diced

½ cup cooked quinoa

2 tablespoons vegetable broth

¼ teaspoon garlic powder

3 tablespoons light cream cheese

12 large button mushrooms, stems removed

4 tablespoons shredded Parmesan cheese

1. Preheat oven to 375°F.
2. Heat oil in a small skillet over medium heat 1 minute. Add onion and bacon and sauté 3–4 minutes until softened. Add quinoa, broth, and garlic powder and cook another 3–4 minutes, stirring frequently. Remove from heat, let cool, and transfer to a small bowl. Stir in cream cheese.
3. Place mushrooms on a large ungreased baking sheet and divide filling among them. Bake 15 minutes until starting to brown.
4. Remove from oven, top with Parmesan cheese, and bake another 2–3 minutes until cheese is melted and lightly toasted. Serve warm or store covered in the refrigerator for up to 3 days.

Honey Raisin Bars

These bars are great for a quick breakfast, afternoon snack, or healthier dessert. If you like chewier cookies or need to cut the fat in your diet, you can substitute applesauce, plums, prunes, or mashed banana for the sunflower oil.

½ cup all-purpose flour

¼ teaspoon baking soda

⅛ teaspoon sea salt

¼ teaspoon ground cinnamon

¾ cup quick-cooking oats

1 large egg white

2½ tablespoons sunflower oil

¼ cup amber honey

¼ cup skim milk

½ teaspoon vanilla extract

½ cup golden raisins

1. Preheat oven to 350°F. Line a 9" × 12" baking sheet with parchment paper.
2. Sift flour, baking soda, salt, and cinnamon together into a large bowl. Stir in oats.
3. In a separate medium bowl, mix egg white, oil, honey, milk, vanilla, and raisins. Add to bowl with dry ingredients and combine.
4. Spread batter in an even layer on prepared baking sheet and bake 15 minutes or to desired crispiness.
5. Cool slightly about 20 minutes, then use a sharp knife or pizza cutter to slice into eighteen equal pieces. Store in an airtight container in the refrigerator for up to 5 days.

SERVES 18	
Per Serving:	
Calories	80
Fat	2g
Saturated Fat	0g
Sodium	40mg
Carbohydrates	13g
Fiber	1g
Sugar	7g
Protein	1g

INDIVIDUAL VERSUS BATCH BAKING

Baking a batch of bar cookies is the simplest way to make cookies. But you can also scoop teaspoons of the batter onto a baking sheet. Bake for 12–15 minutes. (Longer baking time will result in crispier cookies.)

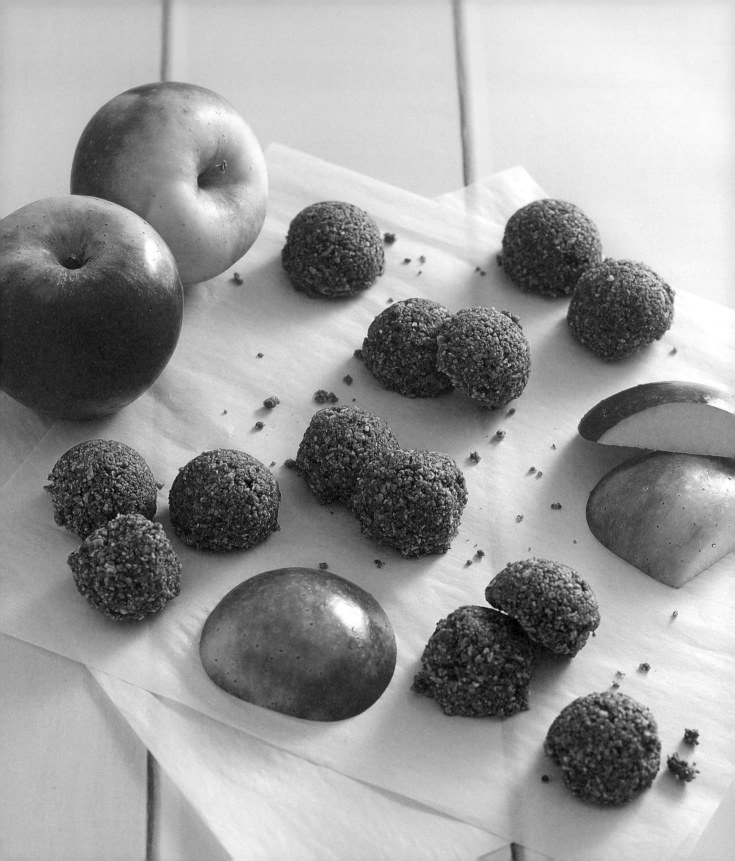

Apple Almond Energy Bites

These grain- and dairy-free bites may be simple to make and require very few ingredients—but they're quite tasty and filling. Enjoy them as a snack or a healthy dessert.

1 cup dried red apple rings (about 15 rings)

½ cup creamy unsalted natural almond butter

½ cup unsweetened grated coconut

1 teaspoon vanilla extract

¼ teaspoon ground cinnamon

⅛ teaspoon salt

1 teaspoon amber honey

1   Line a large baking sheet with parchment paper.
2   Combine all ingredients in a food processor and pulse until mostly smooth.
3   Form dough into fourteen balls and place on prepared baking sheet.
4   Refrigerate until firm, about 1 hour. Serve, or store in an airtight container in the refrigerator for up to 5 days.

SERVES 14	
Per Serving:	
Calories	90
Fat	7g
Saturated Fat	2.5g
Sodium	25mg
Carbohydrates	8g
Fiber	2g
Sugar	5g
Protein	2g

CHAPTER 8

Salads, Dressings, and Sauces

Napa Cabbage Slaw

SERVES 6

Per Serving:

Calories	90
Fat	3g
Saturated Fat	0g
Sodium	170mg
Carbohydrates	11g
Fiber	3g
Sugar	5g
Protein	3g

Serve this simple slaw with Asian-inspired flavors alongside baked or grilled chicken. Or add grilled shrimp or steamed edamame to make it into a meal on its own.

1 small head napa cabbage, cored and thinly sliced

2 large carrots, peeled and shredded

1 cup sliced sugar snap peas

½ large red onion, peeled and chopped

1 tablespoon sesame oil

1 tablespoon low-sodium soy sauce

1 tablespoon Japanese rice wine

1 tablespoon rice wine vinegar

3 tablespoons lemon juice

2 tablespoons lime juice

1 teaspoon minced fresh ginger

1 tablespoon toasted sesame seeds

1 In a large bowl, combine cabbage, carrots, snap peas, and onion.
2 In a separate small bowl, whisk together oil, soy sauce, rice wine, vinegar, lemon juice, lime juice, and ginger. Pour dressing over vegetables and toss to coat.
3 Cover and refrigerate at least 30 minutes. Store leftovers in an airtight container in the refrigerator for up to 2 days. Sprinkle with sesame seeds before serving.

Crunchy Radish and Celery Salad

The crunch and spiciness of radishes liven up this unique salad. Celery and chickpeas provide a nice balance of flavors and textures. When you prep the vegetables, make sure they're all about the same size.

10 medium red radishes, trimmed and chopped

2 large stalks celery, chopped

½ medium white onion, peeled and chopped

1 (15-ounce) can chickpeas, drained and rinsed

1 tablespoon olive oil

3 tablespoons lemon juice

1 tablespoon minced fresh parsley

1 tablespoon minced fresh basil

⅛ teaspoon salt

⅛ teaspoon ground black pepper

1. In a large bowl, combine radishes, celery, onion, and chickpeas.
2. In a separate small bowl, whisk oil, lemon juice, parsley, basil, salt, and pepper. Pour dressing over vegetables and toss to coat. Serve immediately.

SERVES 4	
Per Serving:	
Calories	190
Fat	6g
Saturated Fat	0.5g
Sodium	330mg
Carbohydrates	27g
Fiber	8g
Sugar	6g
Protein	8g

Grapefruit and Beet Salad

SERVES 6

Per Serving:

Calories	90
Fat	0.5g
Saturated Fat	0g
Sodium	95mg
Carbohydrates	20g
Fiber	2g
Sugar	17g
Protein	3g

NUTTY FOR NUTS

With a combination of fat, protein, and fiber, nuts make a satisfying snack or addition to a meal. Research shows that people who consume nuts daily manage their weight better, most likely due to this balance of nutrients.

Sweet, tart, and spicy ingredients make this dish a flavor explosion. Grapefruits are in season during the colder months, so give this pretty salad a try over the holidays.

2 medium beets, trimmed

10 ounces baby arugula

2 large red grapefruits, peeled and sectioned

2 medium red radishes, trimmed and thinly sliced

3 tablespoons red wine vinegar

2 tablespoons amber honey

⅛ teaspoon salt

⅛ teaspoon ground black pepper

2 tablespoons chopped roasted pistachios

1 Preheat oven to 400°F.

2 Wrap beets loosely in foil and place on a large rimmed baking sheet.

3 Roast beets 50 minutes or until a knife can be inserted easily into the center of each beet.

4 Remove from oven, unwrap, and let cool 30 minutes.

5 Rub beets with paper towels to remove skins. Slice thinly.

6 In a large bowl, combine beets, arugula, grapefruit sections, and radishes. In a separate small bowl, whisk together vinegar, honey, salt, and pepper. Pour dressing over salad and toss to coat.

7 Top salad with pistachios before serving.

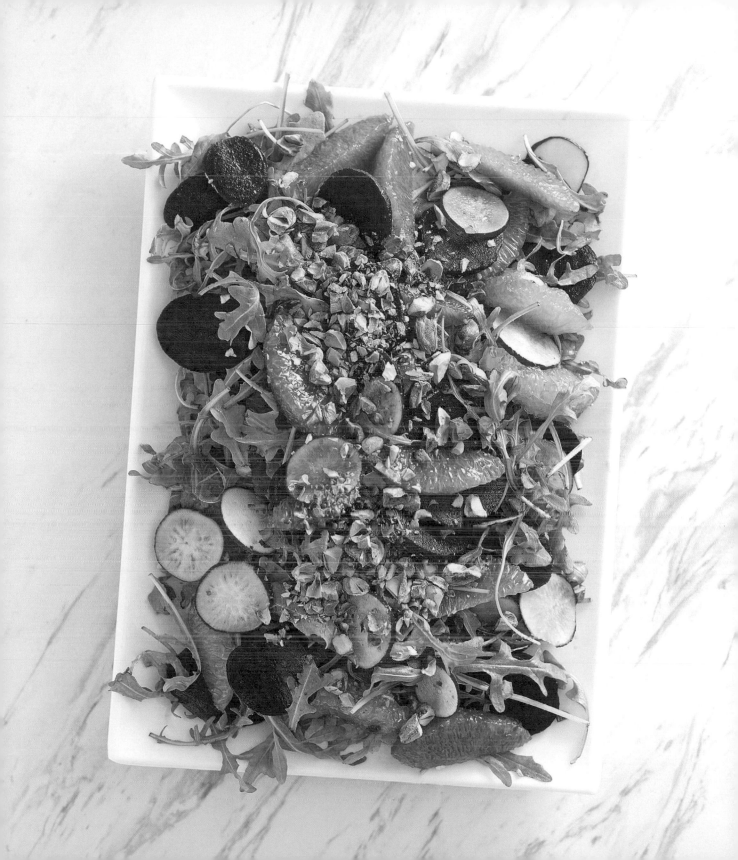

Orange-Avocado Slaw

Per Serving:

Calories	50
Fat	3.5g
Saturated Fat	0g
Sodium	130mg
Carbohydrates	5g
Fiber	1g
Sugar	2g
Protein	2g

CITRUS TO THE RESCUE

Adding a small amount of fresh citrus juice over sliced avocado or guacamole will keep the avocado from browning for at least a day or two. The citric acid in lemon, lime, and orange juice is a potent antioxidant, which works against oxygen to slow down the browning process.

Use this flavorful slaw in place of plain coleslaw as a fresh and tasty side for sandwiches or grilled chicken.

¼ **cup pulp-free orange juice**

½ **teaspoon curry powder**

⅛ **teaspoon ground cumin**

¼ **teaspoon granulated sugar**

1 **teaspoon white wine vinegar**

1 **tablespoon olive oil**

1 **medium ripe avocado, peeled, pitted, and chopped**

5 **cups broccoli slaw mix**

½ **teaspoon sea salt**

¼ **teaspoon ground black pepper**

1   In a small bowl, whisk together orange juice, curry powder, cumin, sugar, and vinegar. Add oil in a steady stream, whisking until emulsified.

2   In a separate large bowl, toss avocado and slaw mix; drizzle with vinaigrette. Refrigerate covered at least 30 minutes.

3   Season with salt and pepper and serve. Store leftovers in an airtight container in the refrigerator for up to 2 days.

Spinach Salad with Pomegranate

Spinach, pomegranates, and walnuts provide rich flavor and healthy antioxidants in this festive salad. Add grilled chicken or fish to make it a delicious main meal.

1 pound fresh spinach, roughly chopped

½ small red onion, peeled and thinly sliced

8 ounces Roma tomatoes, cut into ½" wedges

⅓ cup chopped walnuts

½ teaspoon salt

¼ cup lemon juice

1½ tablespoons olive oil

¼ cup pomegranate seeds

1 Place spinach, onion, tomatoes, and walnuts in a large bowl and toss lightly.

2 In a separate small bowl, whisk together salt, lemon juice, and oil. Drizzle over salad; toss lightly.

3 Garnish salad with pomegranate seeds and serve immediately.

SERVES 6	
Per Serving:	
Calories	110
Fat	8g
Saturated Fat	1g
Sodium	260mg
Carbohydrates	8g
Fiber	3g
Sugar	3g
Protein	4g

THE POWER OF POMEGRANATE

Pomegranate arils are packed with fiber, vitamin C, and potassium. They also contain plant antioxidants called polyphenols, tannins, and anthocyanins that may help decrease risks of chronic diseases like cancer and heart disease.

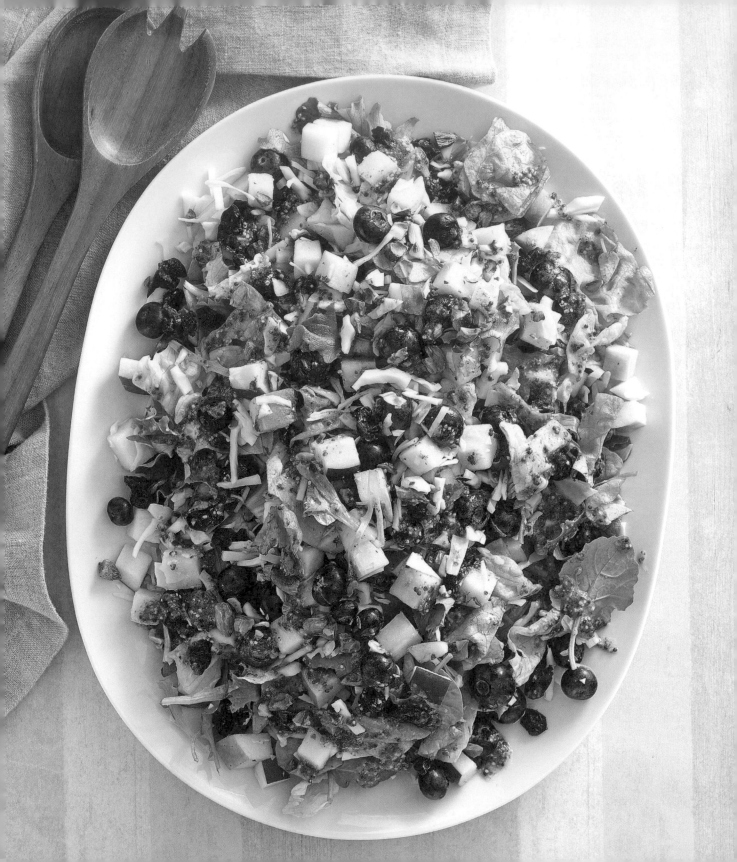

Power Salad

This salad is packed with nutritious superfoods like berries, kale, and nuts. The varied tastes and textures work well together for a hearty and filling lunch or dinner. If you'd like to make it ahead of time, refrigerate the salad and dressing separately and toss together just before serving.

1 (10-ounce) bag shaved Brussels sprouts

1 (5-ounce) package baby kale

6 cups chopped butter lettuce

1 cup fresh blueberries

1 cup chopped red apple

¼ cup dried cranberries

¼ cup chopped pistachios

¼ cup Dijon Vinaigrette (see recipe in this chapter)

Combine Brussels sprouts, kale, lettuce, blueberries, apple, cranberries, and pistachios in a large bowl. Add dressing, toss, and serve.

SERVES 8	
Per Serving:	
Calories	110
Fat	5g
Saturated Fat	0.5g
Sodium	180mg
Carbohydrates	14g
Fiber	3g
Sugar	7g
Protein	3g

Honey-Dijon Tuna Salad

SERVES 2

Per Serving:

Calories	180
Fat	1.5g
Saturated Fat	0g
Sodium	340mg
Carbohydrates	17g
Fiber	2g
Sugar	13g
Protein	25g

This salad is perfect on its own for a light lunch, but you can also turn it into a pasta salad. Just add 1 cup cold cooked pasta shells to the tuna mixture.

1 (5-ounce) can solid white tuna in water, drained

½ cup diced celery

¼ cup diced yellow onion

½ cup diced red bell pepper

¼ cup nonfat plain Greek yogurt

1 teaspoon Dijon mustard

1 teaspoon lemon juice

¼ teaspoon amber honey

2 tablespoons raisins

2 cups tightly packed iceberg lettuce

Use a fork to flake tuna into a medium bowl. Add celery, onion, bell pepper, yogurt, mustard, lemon juice, honey, and raisins and mix well. Serve over lettuce.

Avocado and Peach Salad

The peach and vanilla add sweet flavors that combine well with the savory ingredients in this salad. If you don't have arugula on hand, spinach also works well in this recipe.

2 tablespoons water

2 tablespoons frozen orange juice concentrate

1 clove garlic, peeled and minced

1 teaspoon rice wine vinegar

1 tablespoon extra-virgin olive oil

½ teaspoon vanilla extract

½ teaspoon kosher salt

¼ teaspoon ground black pepper

1½ cups tightly packed baby arugula

2 tablespoons fresh tarragon leaves

1 medium ripe avocado, peeled, pitted, and diced

1 large peach, peeled, pitted, and diced

½ cup thinly sliced Vidalia onion

1 In a large measuring cup, whisk water, orange juice concentrate, garlic, vinegar, oil, vanilla, salt, and pepper together until well mixed.

2 Arrange layers of arugula and tarragon, then avocado, peach, and onion, on a large platter. Drizzle with orange vinaigrette. Serve immediately.

SERVES 4	
Per Serving:	
Calories	140
Fat	9g
Saturated Fat	1g
Sodium	270mg
Carbohydrates	14g
Fiber	3g
Sugar	8g
Protein	3g

EXPERIMENT SENSIBLY

When it comes to new herbs and spices, err on the side of caution. Not sure whether or not you like a seasoning? Mix all other ingredients together and test a bite of salad with a pinch of the herb or spice before adding it to the entire recipe.

Summer Salad

SERVES 6

Per Serving:

Calories	80
Fat	5g
Saturated Fat	0g
Sodium	110mg
Carbohydrates	8g
Fiber	2g
Sugar	4g
Protein	2g

Serve this fresh and colorful salad alongside grilled fish or chicken. To keep the colors bright and vibrant, add the dressing right before serving.

2 cups chopped snap peas

2 cups sliced summer squash

½ cup chopped carrot

3 tablespoons minced button mushrooms

2 cups chopped cucumbers

¼ cup thinly sliced red onion

2 tablespoons canola oil

2 tablespoons balsamic vinegar

¼ teaspoon salt

¼ teaspoon dried thyme

¼ teaspoon ground marjoram

1 Heat 1" water in a large saucepan with a steamer insert over high heat until boiling. Reduce heat to low and place snap peas, squash, carrot, and mushrooms in steamer. Cover and steam 5 minutes.

2 Remove vegetables from steamer with a slotted spoon and transfer to a large bowl. Cover and refrigerate at least 1 hour, up to 2 days.

3 Remove steamed vegetables from refrigerator and add cucumbers and onions.

4 Whisk together oil, vinegar, salt, thyme, and marjoram in a separate small bowl. Pour over vegetables and toss lightly. Serve immediately.

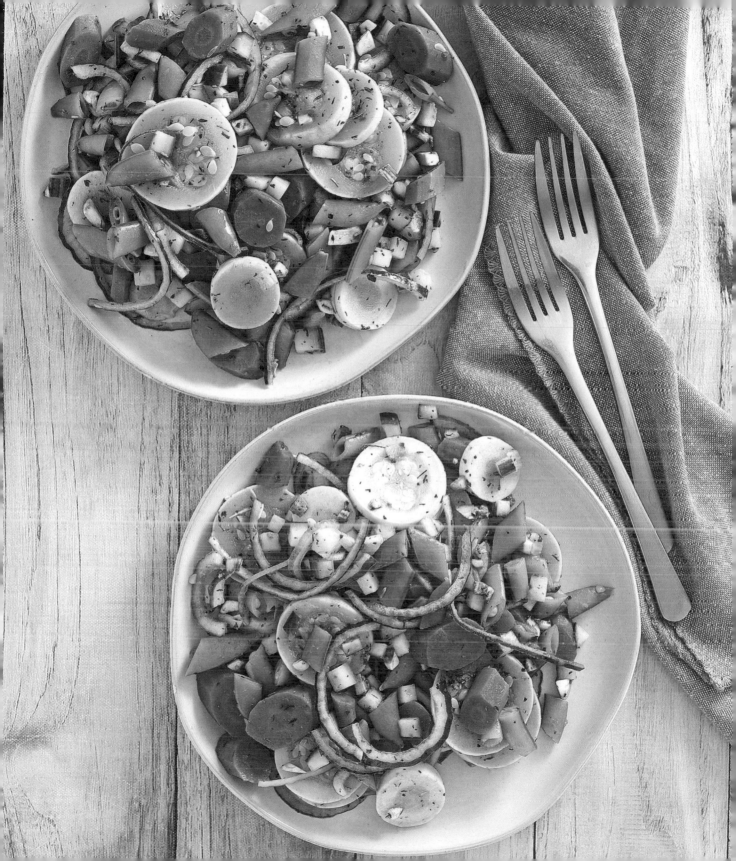

Dijon Vinaigrette

MAKES 5 TABLESPOONS

Per Serving (1 tablespoon):	
Calories	80
Fat	8g
Saturated Fat	1g
Sodium	300mg
Carbohydrates	0g
Fiber	0g
Sugar	0g
Protein	0g

Once you make your own salad dressing, you'll never want to buy bottled dressing again! Use this recipe as a template and make it your own. Try different flavored vinegars, oils, and mustards or add herbs, minced shallots, crushed peppers, or citrus juice.

1 tablespoon Dijon mustard

½ teaspoon sea salt

½ teaspoon ground black pepper

1 tablespoon red wine vinegar

3 tablespoons extra-virgin olive oil

Place all ingredients in a small bowl; use a wire whisk or fork to mix until emulsified. Store leftovers in an airtight container in the refrigerator for up to 1 week.

Quick Tomato Sauce

Ditch the jarred variety; creating a homemade sauce is a cinch with these fresh and simple ingredients. It is great over whole-grain pasta, vegetables, or chicken.

2 tablespoons olive oil

2 cloves garlic, peeled and minced

1 medium yellow onion, peeled and chopped

2 pounds very ripe Roma tomatoes, peeled, seeded, and chopped

2 large sprigs fresh thyme

1 bay leaf

½ teaspoon sea salt

¼ teaspoon ground black pepper

1 tablespoon chopped fresh basil

1 tablespoon chopped fresh oregano

1 tablespoon chopped fresh tarragon

1 Heat oil in a large skillet over medium heat 30 seconds. Add garlic and onion and sauté until fragrant, about 1 minute.

2 Add tomatoes, thyme, bay leaf, salt, and pepper to skillet. Simmer, uncovered, over medium heat, stirring often, until tomatoes are soft and sauce has thickened, about 30 minutes.

3 Discard thyme sprigs and bay leaf. Add basil, oregano, and tarragon before serving. Store leftovers in an airtight container in the refrigerator for up to 4 days.

SERVES 8	
Per Serving:	
Calories	60
Fat	3.5g
Saturated Fat	0.5g
Sodium	150mg
Carbohydrates	6g
Fiber	2g
Sugar	4g
Protein	1g

Pesto Sauce

MAKES 3 CUPS

Per Serving (2 tablespoons):

Calories	160
Fat	17g
Saturated Fat	2.5g
Sodium	115mg
Carbohydrates	2g
Fiber	1g
Sugar	0g
Protein	2g

If you have a lot of basil in your garden, make a double or triple batch of this Pesto Sauce and freeze some for a taste of summer you can enjoy anytime. Freeze a full batch in a tightly sealed container. To freeze small amounts, pour it into ice cube trays and freeze until solid. Once it's frozen, you can place the pesto cubes in zip-top freezer bags for up to 2 months.

¾ cup pine nuts

4 cups tightly packed fresh basil leaves

½ cup grated Parmesan cheese

3 large garlic cloves, peeled

¼ teaspoon salt

1 teaspoon ground black pepper

½ cup extra-virgin olive oil, divided

1 Preheat oven to 350°F.

2 Spread pine nuts on a large ungreased baking sheet. Bake about 5 minutes, then stir. Continue to bake another 10 minutes until nuts are golden brown and highly aromatic, stirring occasionally.

3 Let nuts cool completely, about 30 minutes, and set aside.

4 Fill a medium heavy-bottomed saucepan halfway with water. Place over medium heat and bring to a boil. Next to pot, place a large bowl filled with ice water. Using tongs, dip a few basil leaves into boiling water. Blanch 3 seconds, then place in ice water. Repeat the process until all basil has been blanched, adding more ice to water as needed. Drain blanched basil and pat dry with a towel.

5 In a blender or food processor, combine pine nuts, basil, cheese, garlic, salt, pepper, and all but 1 tablespoon oil; process until smooth and uniform. Pour into an airtight container and pour remaining oil on top to act as a protective barrier. Cover and store in the refrigerator for up to 5 days.

Cucumbers with Minted Yogurt

Serve this fresh cucumber dish alongside your favorite grilled meat or poultry. It can also be used as a condiment to top a sandwich or turkey burger.

1 cup nonfat plain yogurt

1 clove garlic, peeled and finely chopped

¼ teaspoon ground cumin

1 teaspoon lemon zest

½ cup chopped fresh mint

1 tablespoon lemon juice

¼ teaspoon salt

4 cups seeded and chopped cucumbers

1 Combine yogurt, garlic, cumin, lemon zest, mint, lemon juice, and salt in a blender or food processor; blend until smooth.

2 Transfer yogurt mixture to a large bowl and add cucumbers; mix. Refrigerate covered at least 2 hours before serving, up to 2 days.

SERVES 8	
Per Serving:	
Calories	25
Fat	0g
Saturated Fat	0g
Sodium	95mg
Carbohydrates	5g
Fiber	0g
Sugar	3g
Protein	2g

Lemon Almond Dressing

MAKES ⅔ CUP

Per Serving (1 tablespoon):	
Calories	25
Fat	2g
Saturated Fat	0g
Sodium	10mg
Carbohydrates	2g
Fiber	1g
Sugar	1g
Protein	1g

Almonds work as a nice base for this unique dressing that has a terrific blend of lemon, herbs, and ginger.

¼ cup raw almonds

1 tablespoon lemon juice

¼ cup water

1½ teaspoons amber honey

¼ teaspoon lemon pepper

1 (½") piece peeled ginger

¼ clove garlic, peeled

1½ teaspoons chopped fresh chives

1½ teaspoons chopped fresh sweet basil

Put all ingredients in a food processor or blender; process until smooth. Store leftovers in an airtight container in the refrigerator for up to 3 days.

CHAPTER 9

Soups, Stews, and Chilis

Slow Cooker Taco Soup

SERVES 12

Per Serving:

Calories	250
Fat	6g
Saturated Fat	1g
Sodium	520mg
Carbohydrates	32g
Fiber	2g
Sugar	8g
Protein	21g

Serve this soup with tortilla chips, reduced-fat Cheddar cheese, and chopped avocado for a hearty lunch or dinner.

1 tablespoon olive oil

1½ pounds extra-lean ground turkey

2 (28-ounce) cans crushed tomatoes including juice

1 (14-ounce) can black beans, drained and rinsed

1 (14-ounce) can pinto beans, drained and rinsed

1 (14-ounce) can kidney beans, drained and rinsed

1 (14-ounce) can corn kernels, drained and rinsed

2 tablespoons mild taco seasoning

1 Heat oil in a large skillet over medium-high heat 30 seconds. Add turkey and cook 8 minutes or until no longer pink.

2 Transfer turkey to a 4- to 6-quart slow cooker. Add tomatoes, beans, corn, and taco seasoning and stir to combine. Cover and cook on low heat 8 hours, then serve. Store leftovers in an airtight container in the refrigerator for up to 3 days.

Roasted Red Pepper and Pumpkin Soup

Simple, clean ingredients come together to create a flavorful nutritious soup that is low in calories and fat, yet surprisingly filling. Paprika and cayenne give the recipe a nice kick, but you can leave out the cayenne if you like less spice.

5 medium red bell peppers, seeded and quartered

⅓ cup pumpkin purée

3 cups vegetable broth

½ teaspoon smoked paprika

⅛ teaspoon cayenne pepper

½ teaspoon salt

SERVES 4	
Per Serving:	
Calories	70
Fat	0.5g
Saturated Fat	0g
Sodium	700mg
Carbohydrates	13g
Fiber	3g
Sugar	8g
Protein	2g

1 Preheat broiler on high. Line a large baking sheet with parchment paper or spray with nonstick cooking spray.

2 Place peppers on prepared baking sheet. Broil peppers 10 minutes, then turn them over and broil another 8 minutes.

3 Remove sheet from oven and set aside to cool 10 minutes.

4 Add ½ peppers and 2 cups broth to a blender or food processor and blend on high speed 1 minute. Add remaining peppers, pumpkin purée, and broth, paprika, cayenne pepper, and salt. Blend another 2 minutes until smooth.

5 Transfer mixture to a medium saucepan and warm over medium heat 5 minutes until heated through. Serve immediately. Store leftovers in an airtight container in the refrigerator for up to 3 days.

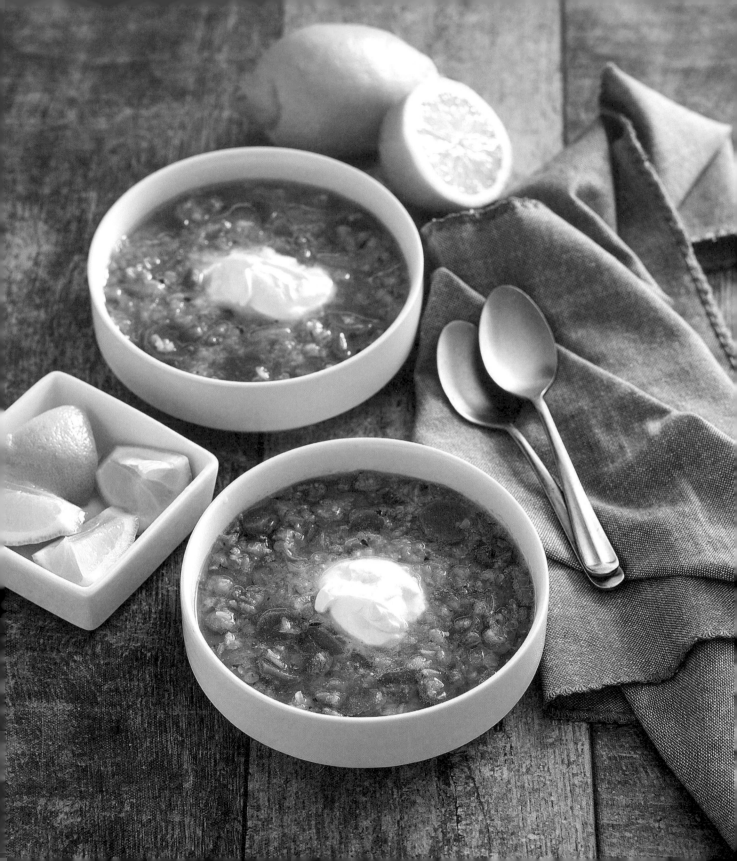

Lentil Soup with Herbs and Lemon

A dollop of low-fat sour cream or nonfat Greek yogurt makes a nice creamy garnish for this savory soup.

1 cup red lentils, covered and soaked overnight in 1 cup water in the refrigerator

6 cups low-sodium chicken broth

2 teaspoons olive oil

1 medium carrot, peeled and chopped

1 stalk celery, sliced

1 medium yellow onion, peeled and chopped finely

1 tablespoon dried tarragon

½ teaspoon dried oregano

½ teaspoon sea salt

¼ teaspoon ground black pepper

1 tablespoon lemon juice

4 thin lemon slices

1 Drain and rinse lentils. Add lentils and broth to a large saucepan over medium heat; bring to a boil. Reduce heat to low and simmer until tender, about 15 minutes.

2 While lentils are cooking, heat oil in a medium skillet over medium-high heat 30 seconds. Add carrot, celery, and onion and sauté 8 minutes, or until onion is golden brown. Remove from heat and set aside.

3 Add vegetables, tarragon, oregano, salt, and pepper to pan with lentils. Cook 2 minutes. Stir in lemon juice.

4 Ladle into serving bowls and garnish with lemon slices. Store leftovers in an airtight container in the refrigerator for up to 3 days.

SERVES 4	
Per Serving:	
Calories	240
Fat	3.5g
Saturated Fat	0g
Sodium	420mg
Carbohydrates	34g
Fiber	8g
Sugar	4g
Protein	17g

WHY SOAK LENTILS?

Soaking lentils overnight helps make them more digestible by neutralizing antinutrients they contain, such as phytic acid. Soaking makes the minerals lentils contain more available to the body.

White Bean and Escarole Soup

SLOW COOKER METHOD

This soup can also be prepared using a slow cooker. Soak beans as described in step 1; drain. Add beans, onion, potato, garlic, Canadian bacon, and 2½ cups water to slow cooker. Cook 8–10 hours on low heat. At end of cooking, add escarole and simmer 5–10 minutes until escarole is wilted and tender, then add salt and pepper.

This hearty, smoky, healthy soup goes great with a slice of whole-grain bread. The savory beans and potatoes are given an extra kick of flavor with the Canadian bacon.

1 cup dried navy beans

1 cup chopped yellow onion

½ cup chopped russet potato

1 clove garlic, peeled and minced

3 ounces Canadian bacon, cut in ½" cubes

2½ cups water

½ teaspoon salt

¼ teaspoon ground black pepper

1 teaspoon vegetable oil

8 ounces escarole, coarsely chopped

1　Place beans and 3 cups water in a medium saucepan over high heat. Bring to a boil, then remove from heat. Cover and allow beans to soak covered, overnight, in the refrigerator.

2　Drain beans and place them in a pressure cooker with onion, potato, garlic, bacon, 2½ cups water, salt, pepper, and oil. Close cover securely, place pressure regulator on vent pipe, and cook 30 minutes with pressure regulator rocking slowly. (If using an electric pressure cooker, follow manufacturer instructions.) Let pressure drop on its own.

3　Add escarole and simmer 5 minutes or until escarole is wilted and tender, then serve. Store leftovers in an airtight container in the refrigerator for up to 3 days.

Cold Roasted Red Pepper Soup

Add a dash of fresh cracked pepper or crushed red pepper to add more "heat" to this refreshing cold soup.

3 large red bell peppers

1 teaspoon olive oil

½ cup chopped yellow onion

3¼ cups low-sodium chicken broth

½ cup nonfat plain yogurt

½ teaspoon sea salt

4 sprigs fresh basil

SERVES 4	
Per Serving:	
Calories	80
Fat	1.5g
Saturated Fat	0g
Sodium	370mg
Carbohydrates	12g
Fiber	3g
Sugar	8g
Protein	5g

1 Preheat broiler on high.

2 Place bell peppers on a large ungreased baking sheet or broiler rack and broil about 2" from heat 15 minutes or until skins are blistered and charred. Turn peppers every 5 minutes while cooking.

3 Place peppers in a large bowl and cover with plastic wrap. Set aside 10 minutes.

4 Remove peppers from bowl. Using a sharp paring knife, remove blackened skins. Cut peppers in half, remove seeds, then roughly chop peppers. Set aside.

5 Heat oil in a medium saucepan over medium-high heat 30 seconds. Add onion and sauté onion 5 minutes or until transparent. Add peppers and broth and bring to a boil.

6 Reduce heat to low and simmer 15 minutes, then remove from heat.

7 Transfer mixture to a blender or food processor and purée until smooth (working in batches if needed).

8 Pour mixture into a large bowl and set aside 30 minutes to cool, then stir in yogurt and salt.

9 Refrigerate covered at least 2 hours, up to 3 days. Garnish with basil before serving.

Broccoli and Whole-Grain Pasta Soup

SERVES 6	
Per Serving:	
Calories	100
Fat	6g
Saturated Fat	2.5g
Sodium	400mg
Carbohydrates	10g
Fiber	2g
Sugar	2g
Protein	6g

Combining a hefty dose of vegetables with a moderate amount of whole-grain pasta keeps the carbs in check and the fiber content high in this hearty soup.

2 slices bacon, cut into 1" pieces

½ cup chopped yellow onion

2 cloves garlic, peeled and minced

1 tablespoon tomato paste

3 cups water

1 cup peeled and cubed eggplant

¾ teaspoon salt

¼ teaspoon ground black pepper

½ teaspoon dried oregano

1 cup broccoli florets

1 cup cooked whole-grain pasta shells

2 tablespoons grated Romano cheese

1 Place bacon, onion, and garlic in a 4-quart soup pot over medium heat. Sauté 6 minutes or until browned.

2 Add tomato paste, water, eggplant, salt, pepper, and oregano to pot. Bring to a boil over high heat, then reduce heat to low and simmer 20 minutes or until eggplant is soft.

3 Add broccoli to pot and simmer 5 minutes until broccoli is tender but still slightly crisp. Stir in cooked pasta.

4 Serve soup immediately with a sprinkling of grated cheese. Store leftovers in an airtight container in the refrigerator for up to 3 days.

Versatile Chicken Vegetable Soup

This soup is great as is, but it can be varied every time you make it. Try one or more of these tasty add-ins: 2 cups raw spinach or a 14.5-ounce can of diced tomatoes (each adds 2 grams of carbs per serving); or a whole-grain starch like 2 cups cooked brown rice, 2 cups cooked whole-wheat pasta, or 3 cups corn kernels (each adds 6 grams of carbs per serving).

1 teaspoon olive oil

2 cups chopped carrots

2 cups chopped celery

1 cup chopped yellow onion

2 cups sliced button mushrooms

3 cups cooked and cubed chicken breast

8 cups low-sodium chicken broth

¼ teaspoon garlic powder

1 teaspoon low-sodium garlic and herb seasoning blend

SERVES 12	
Per Serving:	
Calories	90
Fat	1.5g
Saturated Fat	0g
Sodium	130mg
Carbohydrates	5g
Fiber	1g
Sugar	2g
Protein	12g

1 Heat oil in a large pot over medium heat 30 seconds. Add carrots, celery, and onion and sauté 5 minutes, stirring frequently.

2 Add mushrooms, chicken, and broth and bring to a light boil. Reduce heat to low, add garlic powder and seasoning blend, and simmer 10 minutes or until vegetables are tender, then serve. Store leftovers in an airtight container in the refrigerator for up to 3 days.

Low-Cal Garden Soup

SERVES 8

Per Serving:

Calories	60
Fat	1g
Saturated Fat	0g
Sodium	650mg
Carbohydrates	11g
Fiber	3g
Sugar	6g
Protein	2g

USE BALANCE TO RESET YOUR DIET

Overindulge at dinner last night? Don't use that as permission to stray further from your meal plan the rest of the week. Reset by adding plenty of vegetables and lean protein to your meals and snacks after a high-calorie splurge. This soup is a great option for a reset meal.

Six different vegetables combine with garlic and herbs to create a tasty soup that is very low in calories.

1 teaspoon olive oil

¾ cup chopped white onion

1½ cups chopped celery

1½ cups chopped carrots

1½ cups chopped zucchini

1½ cups cut green beans

½ teaspoon garlic powder

1 teaspoon dried oregano

4 cups low-sodium chicken broth

1 (14-ounce) can stewed tomatoes including juice

¼ cup chopped fresh basil

1 Heat oil in a large pot over medium heat 30 seconds. Add onion, celery, and carrots and sauté until crisp-tender, about 10 minutes.

2 Add zucchini, green beans, garlic powder, oregano, broth, and tomatoes and bring to a light boil. Reduce heat to low and simmer until vegetables are tender, about 10 minutes. Garnish with basil before serving. Store leftovers in an airtight container in the refrigerator for up to 3 days.

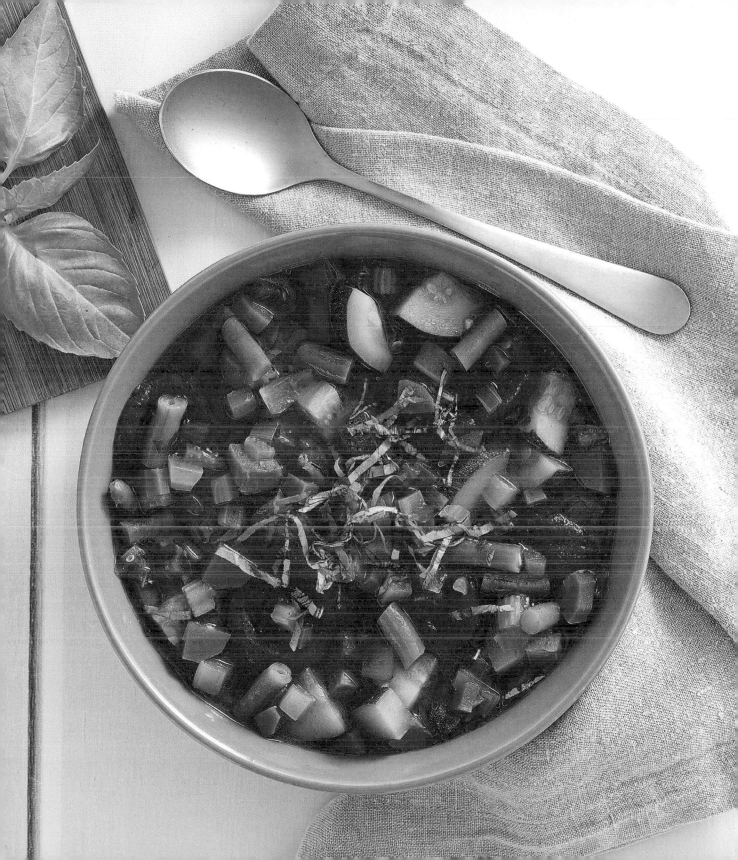

Celery Soup

SERVES 4

Per Serving:

Calories	45
Fat	1.5g
Saturated Fat	0g
Sodium	135mg
Carbohydrates	6g
Fiber	2g
Sugar	2g
Protein	2g

CLEANSING PROPERTIES OF CELERY

In addition to celery containing plenty of fiber, research has revealed compounds in celery have a diuretic effect to get rid of excess body water retention.

This is a simple, clean recipe that you can enhance with your favorite spices. Add a dash of cumin and curry powder for a warm flavor or a pinch of chili powder and crushed red pepper for some heat.

1 teaspoon olive oil, divided

½ cup chopped white onion

1 teaspoon finely chopped garlic

4 cups chopped celery

3 cups low-sodium chicken or vegetable broth

¼ teaspoon ground black pepper

1 Heat ½ teaspoon oil in a large pot over medium heat 30 seconds. Add onion and garlic and sauté until lightly browned, about 3 minutes.

2 Add celery and remaining ½ teaspoon oil to pot and sauté another 5 minutes.

3 Add broth to pot and bring to a boil. Reduce heat to low and simmer 10 minutes or until celery is tender.

4 Remove from heat and let cool 15 minutes, then carefully transfer soup to a food processor or blender in batches and purée until smooth.

5 Return puréed soup to pot and warm on low heat 5 minutes, stirring frequently to prevent thick soup from spattering. Add pepper and serve. Store leftovers in an airtight container in the refrigerator for up to 3 days.

Curried Carrot Soup

This simple soup is made with only a few ingredients, but it is by no means short on taste or unique flavor.

7 cups sliced carrots

1 teaspoon olive oil

½ cup chopped white onion

4 cups low-sodium chicken broth

2 teaspoons curry powder

½ cup light coconut milk

1 Place carrots in a large microwave-safe dish filled with 1" of water. Microwave on high 8 minutes until very tender. Drain and set aside.

2 Heat oil in a medium pot over high heat 30 seconds. Add onion and sauté 2 minutes until almost browned. Add carrots, broth, and curry powder. Heat until almost boiling, about 5 minutes.

3 Remove from heat and let cool 15 minutes, then carefully transfer soup to a food processor or blender in batches and purée until smooth.

4 Return puréed soup to pot, add milk, and warm on low heat 5 minutes, stirring frequently to prevent thick soup from spattering. Store leftovers in an airtight container in the refrigerator for up to 3 days.

SERVES 7	
Per Serving:	
Calories	80
Fat	2g
Saturated Fat	1g
Sodium	135mg
Carbohydrates	14g
Fiber	4g
Sugar	7g
Protein	2g

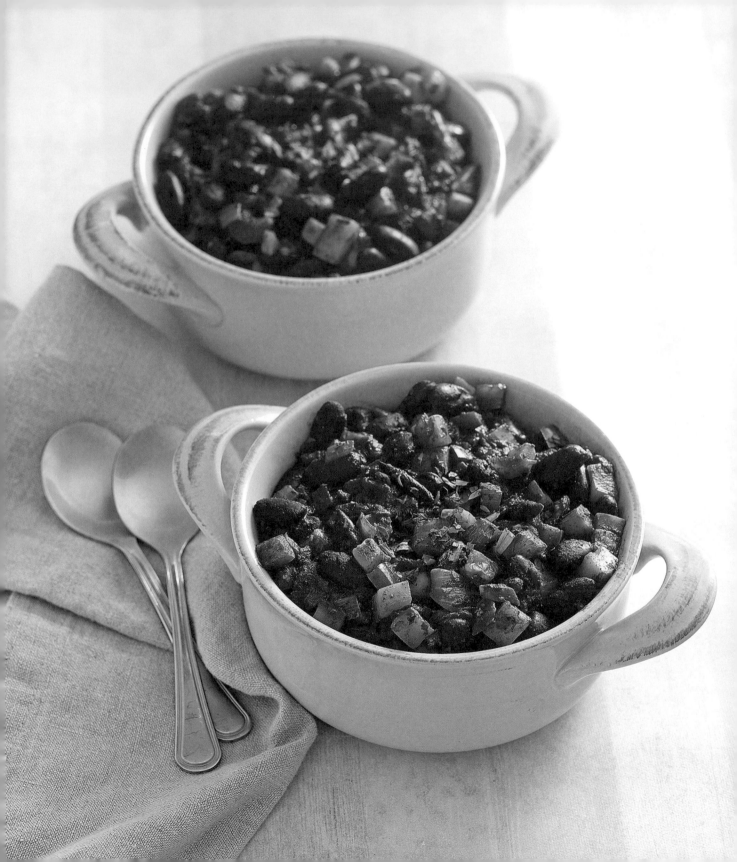

Vegetable and Bean Chili

Warm up with this hearty chili packed with delicious, healthy vegetables. If you like your chili extra-hot, include the seeds from the jalapeño.

4 teaspoons olive oil

2 cups chopped yellow onion

½ cup chopped green bell pepper

3 cloves garlic, peeled and chopped

1 small jalapeño pepper, seeded and finely chopped

1 tablespoon chili powder

1 teaspoon ground cumin

1 (28-ounce) can no-salt-added whole tomatoes, chopped and undrained

2 medium zucchini, peeled and chopped

2 (15-ounce) cans no-salt-added kidney beans, drained and rinsed

1 tablespoon finely chopped semisweet chocolate

3 tablespoons chopped fresh cilantro

1 Heat oil in a large, heavy soup pot over medium-high heat 30 seconds. Add onions, bell pepper, garlic, and jalapeño and sauté until softened, about 5 minutes. Add chili powder and cumin and sauté another 1 minute, stirring frequently to mix well.

2 Add tomatoes with juice and zucchini to pot. Bring to a boil, then reduce heat to medium-low and simmer, partially covered, 15 minutes, stirring occasionally.

3 Stir in beans and chocolate and simmer, stirring occasionally, an additional 5 minutes until beans are heated through and chocolate is melted. Stir in cilantro and serve. Store leftovers in an airtight container in the refrigerator for up to 3 days.

SERVES 8	
Per Serving:	
Calories	160
Fat	3.5g
Saturated Fat	0.5g
Sodium	75mg
Carbohydrates	26g
Fiber	12g
Sugar	7g
Protein	9g

JALAPEÑO SAFETY

The seeds, ribs, and oils of jalapeños can irritate the skin, so it can be useful to wear rubber gloves when handling them. Be sure to wash your hands with soap and water, and avoid touching your eyes, nose, or mouth when working with them.

Eggplant and Tomato Stew

SERVES 4	
Per Serving:	
Calories	130
Fat	2.5g
Saturated Fat	0g
Sodium	65mg
Carbohydrates	23g
Fiber	8g
Sugar	154g
Protein	4g

The hot pepper sauce in this filling and flavorful recipe can be omitted for a less spicy stew. Or you can add a bit more yogurt to counter the heat.

2 medium eggplants, ends trimmed

2 teaspoons olive oil

1 medium Spanish onion, peeled and chopped

1 teaspoon chopped garlic

2 cups chopped canned no-salt-added tomatoes, including juice

1 teaspoon hot pepper sauce

2 tablespoons chopped fresh parsley

¼ cup nonfat plain yogurt

1 Preheat oven to 400°F.

2 Roast whole eggplants on a large ungreased baking sheet until soft, about 45 minutes. Remove from oven and set aside to cool 5 minutes.

3 Cut eggplants in half and scoop the flesh into a medium bowl. Set aside.

4 Heat oil in a large skillet over medium-high heat 30 seconds. Add onion and sauté 5 minutes until softened. Add garlic and sauté 30 seconds. Add eggplant, tomatoes, and pepper sauce.

5 Remove pot from heat and transfer mixture to a food processor. Pulse until mixture becomes creamy.

6 Serve at room temperature. Top each serving with parsley and a dollop of yogurt. Store leftovers in an airtight container in the refrigerator up to 3 days.

Summer Vegetable Stew

Filled with a rainbow of vegetables, this nutritious stew makes the most of fresh summer produce. Serve with whole-grain crackers or toasted wheat bread for a delicious meal.

1 teaspoon olive oil

1 cup chopped turkey sausage

2 cloves garlic, peeled and diced

1 cup chopped white onion

1 cup chopped carrots

1 cup chopped celery

1 cup chopped zucchini

1 cup chopped yellow squash

1 cup chopped green beans

1 cup chopped button mushrooms

1 cup chopped broccoli florets

1 cup chopped red bell pepper

1 cup chopped canned artichokes (water-packed variety)

½ cup corn kernels

1 (14-ounce) can crushed tomatoes including juice

1 (14-ounce) can low-sodium vegetable broth

½ cup canned kidney beans, rinsed

½ cup chopped black olives

¼ cup chopped fresh basil

½ cup grated Parmesan cheese

SERVES 10	
Per Serving:	
Calories	130
Fat	4.5g
Saturated Fat	1.5g
Sodium	410mg
Carbohydrates	16g
Fiber	4g
Sugar	5g
Protein	7g

CUSTOMIZING THIS SOUP

Not a fan of one of the vegetables in this recipe? Double any of ones you like, or substitute 1–2 cups of another, such as cauliflower, eggplant, or spinach. For a vegetarian version, replace the sausage with vegetarian sausage or cubed tofu.

1 Heat oil in a large pot over medium heat 30 seconds. Add sausage, garlic, onion, carrots, and celery and sauté until just tender, about 8 minutes.

2 Add zucchini, yellow squash, green beans, mushrooms, broccoli, bell pepper, artichokes, corn, tomatoes, broth, and kidney beans to pot and bring to a light boil. Reduce heat to low and simmer until vegetables are tender, about 8 minutes.

3 Garnish with olives, basil, and cheese and serve. Store leftovers in an airtight container in the refrigerator for up to 3 days.

Plant-Based Entrées

Baked Broccoli and Tofu

SERVES 6

Per Serving:

Calories	160
Fat	9g
Saturated Fat	1g
Sodium	490mg
Carbohydrates	10g
Fiber	2g
Sugar	3g
Protein	12g

This tasty meatless dinner is cooked together on one sheet pan for less cleanup. Serve it over brown rice for an even heartier meal.

¼ **cup low-sodium soy sauce**

2 tablespoons seasoned rice vinegar

2 tablespoons canola oil

1 teaspoon garlic powder

1 tablespoon sesame seeds

16 ounces extra-firm tofu, cut into ½" cubes

8 cups broccoli florets

1 Preheat oven to 400°F. Line a large baking sheet with parchment paper.
2 In a small bowl, whisk together soy sauce, vinegar, oil, garlic power, and sesame seeds.
3 Place tofu in a separate large bowl, pour in ½ soy sauce mixture, and toss to coat.
4 Spread tofu on one side of prepared baking sheet. Add broccoli to bowl used for tofu, pour in remaining soy sauce mixture, and stir to coat. Spread broccoli on the other half of baking sheet.
5 Bake 15 minutes, turn, and then bake another 8 minutes or until lightly browned. Serve warm.

Cauliflower and Mushroom Taco Filling

This versatile filling can be wrapped in tortillas or lettuce wraps, scooped atop a salad, or served on its own as a delicious side dish. If you like, add beans, cheese, or your favorite meat to pump up the protein.

5 cups chopped cauliflower

1 tablespoon olive oil

4 cups chopped portobello mushrooms

1 cup chopped white onion

½ tablespoon chili powder

½ tablespoon ground cumin

SERVES 5	
Per Serving:	
Calories	80
Fat	3.5g
Saturated Fat	0.5g
Sodium	75mg
Carbohydrates	12g
Fiber	4g
Sugar	5g
Protein	4g

1 Pour 1" water into bottom of a large microwave-safe baking dish. Add cauliflower, cover, and microwave on high 4 minutes. Drain and set aside.

2 Heat oil in a large skillet over medium heat 30 seconds. Add mushrooms and onion and sauté until lightly browned, about 5 minutes.

3 Add cauliflower, chili powder, and cumin to skillet. Stir to distribute spices. Cook, stirring occasionally, 5 minutes until lightly browned and tender.

Portobello Mexican Pizzas

Using large portobello mushrooms instead of crusts cuts the carbo-hydrates and increases the fiber in these tasty pizzas.

SERVES 6	
Per Serving:	
Calories	190
Fat	4.5g
Saturated Fat	2g
Sodium	300mg
Carbohydrates	27g
Fiber	4g
Sugar	7g
Protein	12g

STORING AND PREPARING MUSHROOMS

Do not wash mushrooms until ready to use. If you are serving mushrooms raw, wipe them with a damp cloth rather than washing with water to keep them crisp.

6 large portobello mushrooms (about 4"–5" in diameter), stems removed

1 teaspoon olive oil

1 cup diced white onion

2 cups chopped red bell pepper

1 (15-ounce) can black beans, drained and rinsed well

1 cup corn kernels

½ cup canned diced tomatoes including juice

1 tablespoon ground cumin

2 teaspoons chili powder

¼ teaspoon garlic powder

¾ cup shredded reduced-fat Cheddar cheese

2 tablespoons chopped fresh cilantro

1 Preheat oven to 350°F. Spray a large baking sheet with nonstick cooking spray.

2 Place mushrooms on prepared baking sheet, stem-side up. Bake 15 minutes.

3 While mushrooms are baking, heat oil in a medium skillet over medium heat 30 seconds. Add onion and bell pepper and sauté 5 minutes until lightly browned and tender. Add beans, corn, tomatoes, cumin, chili powder, and garlic powder and heat another 6 minutes, stirring occasionally. Set aside.

4 Remove mushrooms from oven and drain any excess moisture. Stuff each mushroom with ½ cup filling and return to baking sheet.

5 Bake filled mushrooms 15 minutes. Remove from oven, sprinkle each with 2 tablespoons cheese, and bake another 2 minutes until cheese is slightly melted. Garnish with cilantro and serve.

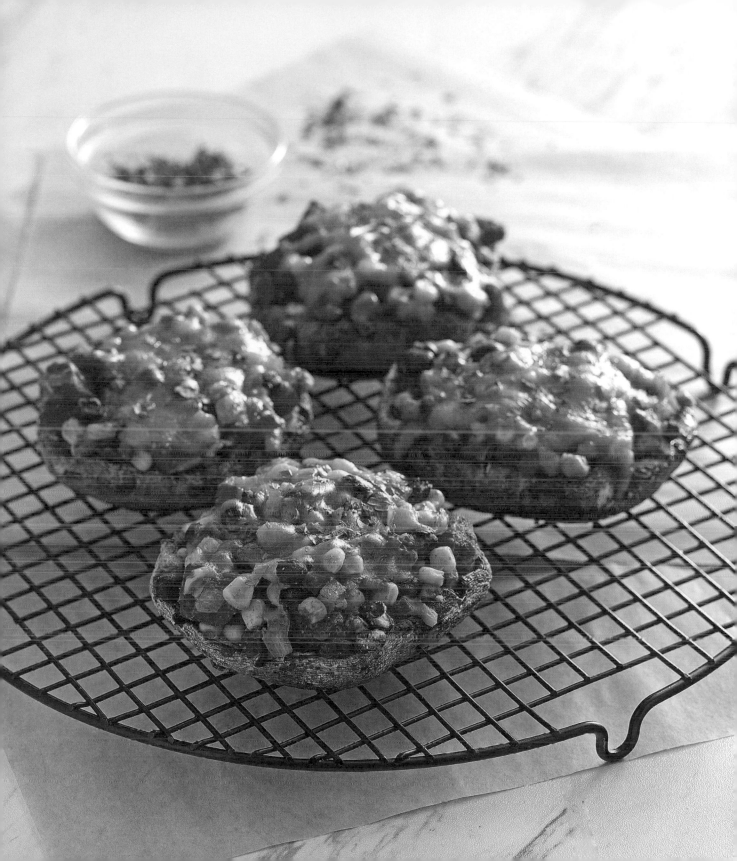

Oven-Roasted Ratatouille

SERVES 12

Per Serving:

Calories	110
Fat	6g
Saturated Fat	1.5g
Sodium	330mg
Carbohydrates	11g
Fiber	2g
Sugar	4g
Protein	2g

A VERSATILE DISH

Ratatouille can be dished up a variety of ways, hot or cold, by itself or topped with egg or low-fat cheese. It can also be served atop salads, scooped inside a pita, or with whole-grain pasta.

Ratatouille, a traditional vegetable dish from France, can be served as a main dish or as a side with your favorite protein.

5 cups peeled and diced eggplant

3 cups diced yellow squash

½ pound green beans, trimmed

½ cup chopped celery

1 cup chopped red onion

4 cloves garlic, peeled and chopped

1 (28-ounce) can diced tomatoes including juice

1 tablespoon chopped fresh parsley

¼ teaspoon salt

½ teaspoon dried rosemary

½ teaspoon dried thyme

¼ cup olive oil

2 tablespoons balsamic vinegar

1 Preheat oven to 375°F.
2 In a large Dutch oven or 9" × 13" baking dish, combine eggplant, squash, green beans, celery, onion, garlic, tomatoes, parsley, salt, rosemary, thyme, and oil.
3 Roast, uncovered, 30 minutes. Stir, then continue roasting another 30 minutes or until vegetables are softened and lightly browned on top.
4 Remove from oven. Stir in balsamic vinegar and serve.

Layered Vegetable Casserole

If you'd like more tomato flavor, top this vegetable-rich dish with your favorite tomato sauce and a dash of black pepper.

1 (10-ounce) package frozen mixed vegetables (corn, peas, carrots, and green beans), thawed

½ cup diced yellow onion

½ cup diced green bell pepper

1 cup no-salt-added tomato juice

⅛ teaspoon celery seed

⅛ teaspoon dried basil

⅛ teaspoon dried oregano

⅛ teaspoon dried parsley

¼ teaspoon garlic powder

3 tablespoons grated Parmesan cheese, divided

1 Preheat oven to 350°F. Spray a large baking dish with nonstick cooking spray.

2 Layer mixed vegetables, onion, and bell pepper in prepared baking dish.

3 In a large glass measuring cup, mix tomato juice, celery seed, basil, oregano, parsley, garlic powder, and 2 tablespoons cheese; pour over vegetables.

4 Cover dish and bake 1 hour.

5 Uncover baking dish and sprinkle with remaining cheese. Continue to bake 10 minutes, or until liquid thickens and mixture bubbles. Serve.

SERVES 4	
Per Serving:	
Calories	90
Fat	1.5g
Saturated Fat	0.5g
Sodium	110mg
Carbohydrates	1.5g
Fiber	1g
Sugar	3g
Protein	4g

SEASON FIRST

When readying vegetables for steaming, add fresh or dried herbs, spices, sliced or diced onions, minced garlic, grated ginger, or any other seasoning you'd normally use. Seasonings will cook into vegetables during steaming.

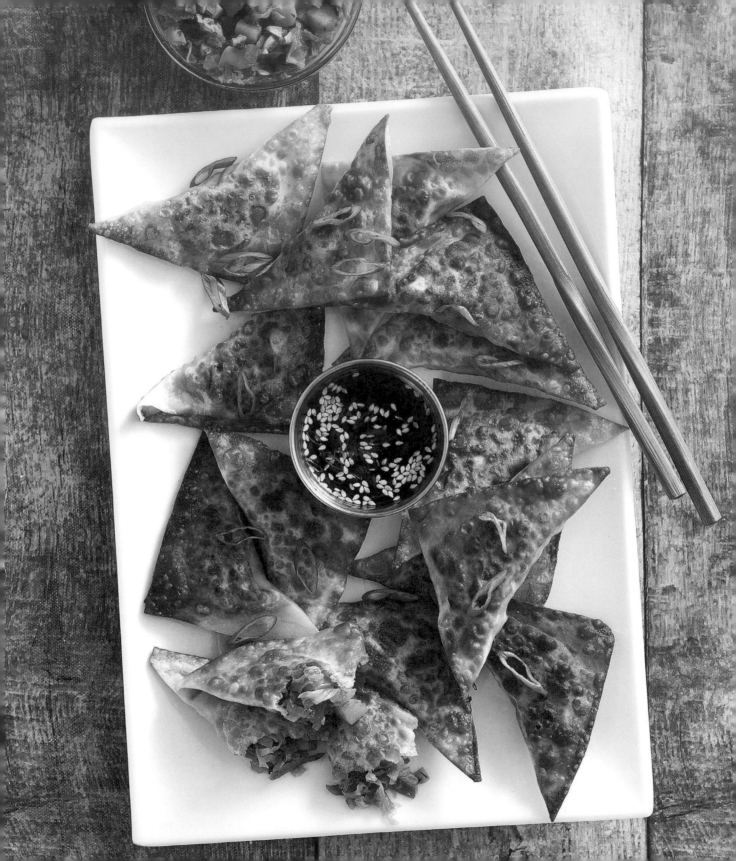

Vegetable Pot Stickers

For softer pot stickers, you can steam them for a few minutes on each side in a covered skillet filled with ¼"–½" of boiling water. Or bake them on a baking sheet at 350°F for about 7–10 minutes per side.

1 tablespoon plus 1 teaspoon sesame oil, divided

1 clove garlic, peeled and finely chopped

1 teaspoon finely chopped fresh ginger

¼ cup chopped scallions

½ cup chopped celery

½ cup shredded carrots

½ cup chopped water chestnuts, drained and rinsed

1 tablespoon low-sodium soy sauce

1 cup chopped napa cabbage

½ cup chopped button mushrooms

12 wonton wrappers

SERVES 12	
Per Serving:	
Calories	45
Fat	1.5g
Saturated Fat	0g
Sodium	100mg
Carbohydrates	6g
Fiber	0g
Sugar	0g
Protein	1g

1 Heat 1 tablespoon oil in a large skillet or wok over medium-high heat 30 seconds; add garlic, ginger, and scallions and sauté a few minutes until slightly browned. Add celery, carrots, and water chestnuts and sauté another 4 minutes.

2 Add soy sauce, cabbage, and mushrooms and sauté 4 minutes until vegetables are slightly softened. Transfer mixture to a large bowl and let cool a few minutes.

3 Lay out wrappers on a clean cutting board. Spoon 1 heaping tablespoon of vegetable mixture onto one side of each wrapper. Wet all edges with water (using your fingers), fold over wrapper to make a triangle, and pinch closed all along edges.

4 Heat remaining 1 teaspoon oil in skillet over high heat and add filled wontons; heat about 4 minutes on each side until lightly browned and slightly crispy. Serve.

Spaghetti Squash and Vegetable Mix

SERVES 6

Per Serving:

Calories	120
Fat	7g
Saturated Fat	1.5g
Sodium	160mg
Carbohydrates	5g
Fiber	2g
Sugar	8g
Protein	4g

Spaghetti squash is a wonderful alternative to pasta because it is packed with vitamins, minerals, and fiber. While it has a consistency similar to spaghetti, it is much lower in carbohydrates; 1 cup of cooked spaghetti squash has 15 grams of carbohydrates, while 1 cup of cooked spaghetti has approximately 45 grams!

1 (2-pound) spaghetti squash, halved and seeded

1 cup frozen peas, thawed

2 tablespoons vegan margarine, melted

8 ounces cherry tomatoes, halved

2 tablespoons grated Romano cheese

¼ teaspoon ground black pepper

1 Preheat oven to 400°F. Spray a 9" × 13" baking dish with nonstick cooking spray.

2 Place squash halves facedown in prepared baking dish. Bake 45 minutes or until squash is tender when pierced with a knife.

3 Remove squash from oven and set aside to cool 10 minutes. Once cooled, flip squash over and use a fork to scoop out cooked squash from outer shell. Scoop into a medium microwave-safe bowl.

4 Add peas and margarine to the bowl with squash; mix well. Cover bowl and place in microwave; cook on high 3 minutes.

5 Top squash with tomatoes, cheese, and pepper before serving.

Chock-Full o' Vegetables Chili

Make this delicious chili even better by sprinkling with chopped chives. Use it as a topping on a baked sweet potato for a delicious treat.

1 (28-ounce) can crushed tomatoes including juice

2 (15-ounce) cans black beans, drained and rinsed

1 (15-ounce) can kidney beans, drained and rinsed

3½ cups sliced cremini mushrooms

2½ cups shredded carrots

2 cups cubed yellow squash

2 cups chopped yellow onions

1 cup chopped red bell pepper

1 cup chopped yellow bell pepper

1 cup chopped orange bell pepper

1 cup finely diced Anaheim chili peppers

3 tablespoons chili powder

1 tablespoon paprika

1 teaspoon minced garlic

1   Combine tomatoes, beans, mushrooms, carrots, squash, onions, and bell peppers in a large pot over high heat. Cook 15 minutes uncovered, stirring occasionally.

2   Add chili peppers, chili powder, paprika, and garlic to pot. Reduce heat to medium-high and continue to cook uncovered another 15 minutes, stirring occasionally.

3   Reduce heat to low, cover pot, and simmer, stirring occasionally, until vegetables are tender, about 25 minutes. Serve. Store leftovers in an airtight container in the refrigerator for up to 3 days.

SERVES 12	
Per Serving:	
Calories	180
Fat	2g
Saturated Fat	0.5g
Sodium	360mg
Carbohydrates	33g
Fiber	6g
Sugar	8g
Protein	11g

WHAT ARE ANAHEIM CHILI PEPPERS?

Anaheim chili peppers are a versatile, mild-flavored pepper. They originated in New Mexico (where they're called *New Mexico chilies*) and became popular in the United States after farmers in California began growing them in the late 1800s.

Sesame Noodle Stir-Fry

SERVES 6

Per Serving:

Calories	120
Fat	6g
Saturated Fat	1g
Sodium	230mg
Carbohydrates	13g
Fiber	3g
Sugar	4g
Protein	6g

STIR-FRY SWAPS

If you don't care for one or more of the vegetables in this recipe, you can substitute a cup of another chopped vegetable of your choice such as broccoli, carrots, and water chestnuts, as long as there are 7 cups of raw vegetables total.

This dish is generally served hot, but you can enjoy leftovers cold with a dash of extra soy sauce and rice vinegar to dress it up.

1 tablespoon plus 1 teaspoon sesame oil, divided

1 cup diced yellow onion

1 cup diced celery

2 cups chopped button mushrooms

1 cup chopped red bell pepper

1 cup diced eggplant

1 cup snap peas

½ teaspoon minced garlic

4 ounces dried soba noodles, cooked

¼ cup chopped unsalted peanuts

½ cup chopped fresh basil

2 tablespoons low-sodium soy sauce

¼ teaspoon crushed red pepper flakes

1 Heat 1 tablespoon oil in a large skillet over medium heat 30 seconds. Add onion, celery, mushrooms, bell pepper, eggplant, and snap peas and sauté 5 minutes.

2 Add garlic to skillet and continue sautéing another 5 minutes or until vegetables are slightly tender.

3 Add noodles to skillet. Stir in remaining oil, peanuts, and basil and warm another 3 minutes.

4 Top with soy sauce and red pepper flakes and serve.

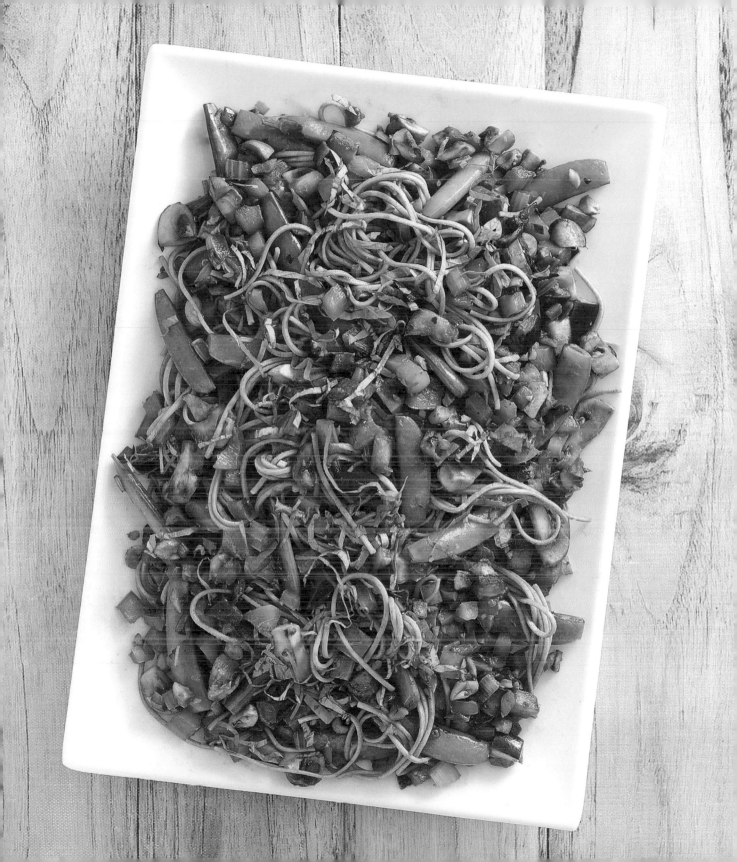

Edamame Succotash

SERVES 7

Per Serving:

Calories	110
Fat	5g
Saturated Fat	0g
Sodium	220mg
Carbohydrates	11g
Fiber	3g
Sugar	2g
Protein	6g

Succotash, a classic American salad, is usually made with lima beans. This version swaps the limas for sweet, nutty soybeans, but feel free to use lima beans if you prefer.

2 tablespoons vegan margarine, divided

2 tablespoons diced red onion

1 cup chopped red bell pepper

1 cup corn kernels

2 cups shelled and cooked edamame

½ teaspoon salt

½ teaspoon ground black pepper

1 Melt 1 tablespoon margarine in a large skillet over medium heat, then add onion and bell pepper. Sauté until slightly tender, about 5 minutes.

2 Add corn, edamame, and remaining margarine to skillet and sauté another 6 minutes. Season with salt and pepper and serve.

Parmesan-Crusted Eggplant

This is a simple way to try out eggplant if you haven't cooked with it before. Serve with Herbed Quinoa with Sun-Dried Tomatoes or Greens in Garlic with Pasta (see recipes in Chapter 13).

1 large eggplant, ends trimmed, sliced lengthwise into ¼" slices

2 teaspoons salt

1 large egg

1 large egg white

½ cup grated Parmesan cheese

3 teaspoons olive oil

SERVES 4	
Per Serving:	
Calories	130
Fat	8g
Saturated Fat	2.5g
Sodium	710mg
Carbohydrates	10g
Fiber	4g
Sugar	4g
Protein	7g

1 Place sliced eggplant in a colander. Sprinkle with salt on both sides and set aside 15 minutes. Rinse eggplant and pat dry with paper towels.

2 In a medium shallow bowl, beat egg and egg white together lightly. Place cheese in a separate medium shallow bowl.

3 Heat oil in a large skillet over medium heat 30 seconds. Dredge eggplant slices in egg and then cheese. In batches, place coated slices in skillet and cook 3 minutes per side or until lightly browned. Serve immediately.

CHAPTER 11

Poultry, Beef, and Pork

Honey and Cider–Glazed Chicken

Citrus and vinegar add fresh flavor and keep this chicken moist—without added fat! Add a side salad to round out the meal.

SERVES 4

Per Serving:

Calories	210
Fat	4.5g
Saturated Fat	1g
Sodium	160mg
Carbohydrates	2g
Fiber	0g
Sugar	2g
Protein	38g

WHY TAKE A REST?

Letting meat and poultry rest for at least 5 minutes after cooking allows it to better hold on to the juices and seal in the moisture for the best flavor and mouthfeel.

3 tablespoons apple cider vinegar

½ teaspoon amber honey

1 teaspoon lemon juice

1 teaspoon Bragg Liquid Aminos

½ teaspoon grated lemon zest

4 (6-ounce) boneless, skinless chicken breasts

1 Preheat oven to 375°F.

2 Combine all ingredients except chicken in a large microwave-safe bowl; microwave on high 30 seconds. Stir until honey is dissolved.

3 Arrange chicken on a rack placed in a medium roasting or broiling pan. Brush or spoon 1 teaspoon glaze over top of each piece. Bake 30 minutes, basting halfway through cooking time, and again 5 minutes before chicken is done.

4 Allow chicken to rest 5 minutes before cutting and serving.

Chicken Breasts in Balsamic Vinegar Sauce

Serve this tangy chicken over your favorite greens or with a vegetable side for a low-carbohydrate, low-calorie meal.

4 (4-ounce) boneless, skinless chicken breasts

¼ teaspoon salt

¼ teaspoon ground black pepper

1 tablespoon salted butter

1 tablespoon olive oil

¼ cup chopped red onion

2 teaspoons minced garlic

3 tablespoons balsamic vinegar

1½ cups low-sodium chicken broth

1 teaspoon dried oregano

SERVES 4	
Per Serving:	
Calories	210
Fat	9g
Saturated Fat	3g
Sodium	230mg
Carbohydrates	4g
Fiber	0g
Sugar	2g
Protein	27g

1 Sprinkle chicken with salt and pepper.

2 Heat butter and oil in a large skillet over medium heat 30 seconds. Add chicken and cook until browned, about 5 minutes on each side. Reduce heat to low and cook another 12 minutes.

3 Transfer chicken to a platter; cover and keep warm.

4 Add onion and garlic to skillet and sauté over medium heat 3 minutes, scraping up browned bits. Add vinegar and bring to a boil. Boil 3 minutes or until reduced to a glaze, stirring constantly.

5 Add chicken broth to skillet and boil until reduced to about ¾ cup liquid. Remove sauce from heat and add oregano.

6 Spoon sauce over chicken and serve immediately.

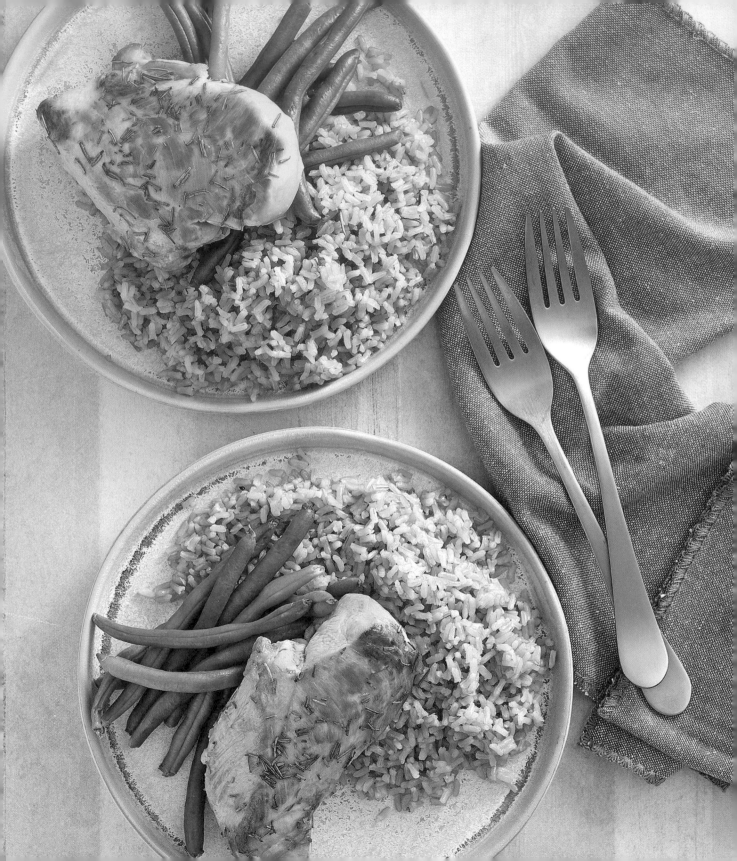

Herbed Chicken and Brown Rice

Brown rice adds fiber, and chicken breasts provide lean protein to this satisfying dish. Add a steamed green vegetable for a well-rounded meal.

1 tablespoon canola oil

4 (4-ounce) boneless, skinless chicken breasts

1 teaspoon garlic powder, divided

1 teaspoon crushed dried rosemary, divided

1 (10.5-ounce) can low-sodium chicken broth

⅓ cup water

2 cups uncooked instant brown rice

SERVES 4

Per Serving:

Calories	360
Fat	8g
Saturated Fat	1g
Sodium	75mg
Carbohydrates	40g
Fiber	2g
Sugar	0g
Protein	30g

1 Heat oil in a large nonstick skillet over medium-high heat 30 seconds. Add chicken and sprinkle with ½ teaspoon each garlic powder and rosemary. Cover and cook 4 minutes on each side or until cooked through (no longer pink in the center).

2 Remove chicken from skillet and set aside.

3 Add broth and water to skillet; stir to deglaze pan and bring to a boil. Stir in rice and remaining garlic powder and rosemary. Return chicken to skillet, cover, and cook on low heat 5 minutes.

4 Remove skillet from heat and let stand, covered, 5 minutes before serving.

Cornflake Chicken

SERVES 4

Per Serving:

Calories	330
Fat	3.5g
Saturated Fat	1g
Sodium	370mg
Carbohydrates	45g
Fiber	0g
Sugar	4g
Protein	31g

Crunchy cornflakes add a great flavor and texture to this chicken. Cut the breasts into strips to serve over a salad or dip into your favorite barbecue sauce.

2 cups crushed cornflakes

⅛ teaspoon salt

⅛ teaspoon ground black pepper

¼ cup liquid egg whites

2 tablespoons buttermilk

4 (4-ounce) boneless, skinless chicken breasts

1 Preheat oven to 425°F. Spray a large baking sheet with nonstick cooking spray.
2 Combine cornflake crumbs, salt, and pepper in a medium shallow bowl.
3 Beat egg whites and buttermilk together in another medium shallow bowl.
4 Dip each chicken breast in egg mixture and then coat in crumb mixture. Place coated chicken on prepared baking sheet and bake 13 minutes. Flip breasts and bake another 13 minutes until no longer pink in the center. Serve.

Spicy Turkey Burgers

With all the spicy flavors, you'll never miss the salt in these burgers. The Cajun spices and jalapeños really give them a kick. Adding some sliced avocado before serving will mellow out the heat.

1 pound ground turkey

¼ cup dried bread crumbs

1 tablespoon salt-free Cajun spice blend

1 large egg

1 tablespoon finely chopped fresh cilantro

2 teaspoons minced jalapeño pepper

1 Preheat a gas or charcoal grill to high heat. Spray grate with non-stick cooking spray.

2 Combine all ingredients in a large bowl. Shape mixture into 4 patties.

3 Grill burgers 6 minutes on each side, or until cooked through (no longer pink in the center). Serve immediately.

SERVES 4

Per Serving:

Calories	200
Fat	10g
Saturated Fat	2g
Sodium	140mg
Carbohydrates	6g
Fiber	0g
Sugar	0g
Protein	27g

PROPER POULTRY AND MEAT HANDLING

Be sure to wash any utensil that comes in contact with raw poultry in hot, soapy water and rinse well. This includes washing any utensil each time it's used to baste, in grilling and roasting, or when baking poultry.

Chipotle Chicken Wraps

SERVES 4

Per Serving:

Calories	240
Fat	7g
Saturated Fat	2.5g
Sodium	390mg
Carbohydrates	21g
Fiber	0g
Sugar	2g
Protein	23g

WHAT IS CHIPOTLE?

A chipotle is a smoke-dried jalapeño chili used in Mexican and Tex-Mex dishes. You can purchase dried chipotle peppers or a seasoning mix with chipotle peppers added. Dash Southwest Chipotle Seasoning Blend is salt-free!

To cut the carbohydrates even more, you can serve this chicken in lettuce wraps or over mixed greens instead of the tortillas.

12 ounces boneless, skinless chicken breast, cut into ½" strips

1 tablespoon lime juice

1 tablespoon olive oil

1 teaspoon chipotle seasoning

⅛ teaspoon ground black pepper

4 (6") whole-wheat tortillas

½ cup mild salsa

1 cup chopped iceberg lettuce

1 Place chicken, lime juice, oil, chipotle seasoning, and pepper in a large shallow dish; mix well. Cover and marinate 1 hour in refrigerator.

2 Preheat oven to 350°F.

3 Wrap tortillas in foil and place on oven rack to heat while cooking chicken.

4 Cook chicken strips 8 minutes until done, turning strips once during cooking.

5 Remove tortillas from oven and unwrap. Place each tortilla on a plate and top with chicken, salsa, and lettuce. Roll tortilla into a burrito shape and serve.

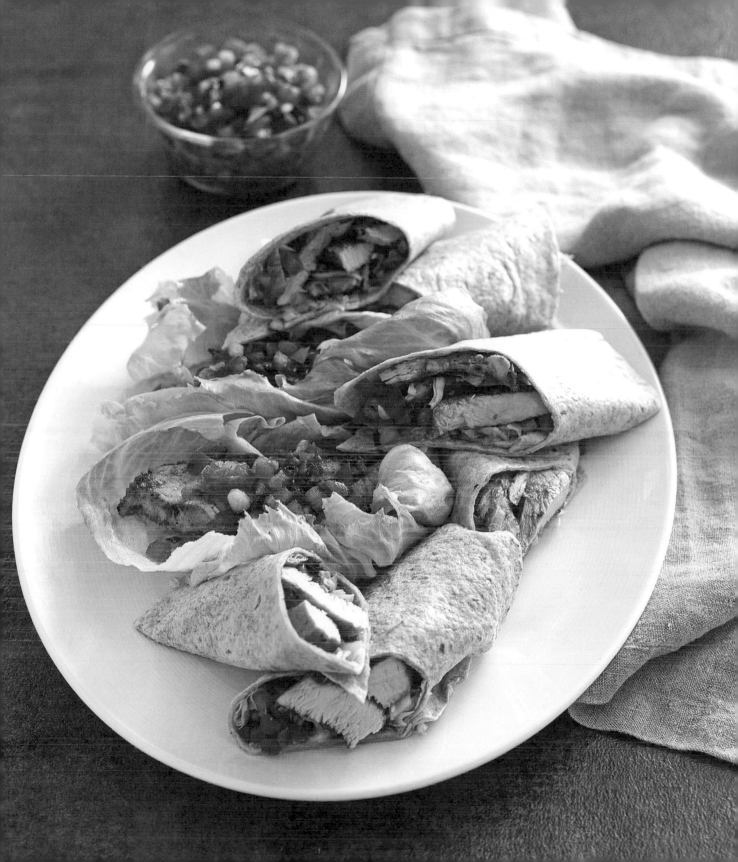

Turkey Chili

SERVES 6	
Per Serving:	
Calories	280
Fat	8g
Saturated Fat	1.5g
Sodium	750mg
Carbohydrates	36g
Fiber	9g
Sugar	14g
Protein	25g

You'll need only about 15 minutes of hands-on time for this easy chili. Then let it simmer for a few hours. Your kitchen will be filled with the enticing aroma of a warm, comforting Tex-Mex dinner.

1 teaspoon olive oil

1 pound lean ground turkey

1 cup chopped white onion

½ cup chopped green bell pepper

2 teaspoons minced garlic

2 (28-ounce) cans crushed tomatoes including juice

1 cup canned black beans, drained and rinsed

1 cup canned red kidney beans, drained and rinsed

3 tablespoons chili powder

1 tablespoon ground cumin

1 teaspoon crushed red pepper

⅛ teaspoon Tabasco sauce

1 Add oil to a large Dutch oven or soup pot. Add turkey and brown over medium-high heat, about 6 minutes.
2 Add onion, bell pepper, and garlic to Dutch oven or pot. Continue cooking until onion is translucent, about 5 minutes.
3 Add tomatoes, beans, chili powder, cumin, red pepper, and Tabasco sauce; bring to a slow boil. Reduce heat to low, cover, and simmer 3 hours before serving, stirring occasionally.

Garden Turkey Meatloaf

Use any of your favorite vegetables in this meatloaf; just chop them all finely and make sure they add up to 1 cup. You can also replace the Cajun seasoning with 1–2 teaspoons of two or more of these seasonings: garlic powder, oregano, paprika, chili powder, or ground black pepper.

1 pound lean ground turkey

½ cup old-fashioned rolled oats

¼ cup finely chopped yellow onion

¼ cup finely chopped button mushrooms

¼ cup finely chopped zucchini

¼ cup finely chopped carrot

½ cup tomato sauce

2 large egg whites

1 teaspoon Cajun seasoning

1 Preheat oven to 350°F. Spray a 5" x 9" loaf pan with nonstick cooking spray.

2 In a large bowl, mix together all ingredients. Transfer to prepared pan.

3 Bake meatloaf 1 hour until no longer pink in the center and an instant-read thermometer registers at least 165°F. Serve.

SERVES 8	
Per Serving:	
Calories	110
Fat	4.5g
Saturated Fat	1g
Sodium	120mg
Carbohydrates	7g
Fiber	1g
Sugar	1g
Protein	14g

WHICH MEAT THERMOMETER IS BEST?

Regular meat thermometers have oven-safe gauges protected by stainless steel, so they can be inserted into a large cut of meat and left in during cooking. Instant-read thermometers provide an immediate display of the food temperature within a minute. The temperature gauge is usually covered in plastic and shouldn't be used in the oven. This type of thermometer is best used for meatloaves and smaller cuts of meat, like chicken parts, pork chops, and fish or beef steaks.

Easy Oven Beef Burgundy

SERVES 4

Per Serving:

Calories	220
Fat	7g
Saturated Fat	3g
Sodium	370mg
Carbohydrates	13g
Fiber	2g
Sugar	5g
Protein	26g

THE DUTCH OVEN DIFFERENCE

Dutch ovens are much more than baking dishes. They can be used on the stovetop, as well as in the oven. Most are made of enameled cast iron and come in an assortment of colors. They can be used for many cooking tasks like sautéing vegetables, braising meat, cooking soups and stews, and even baking bread!

Baking Beef Burgundy in the oven is the simplest way to make this classic dish. Serve it with ½ cup whole-grain pasta or brown rice. For a lower-carbohydrate option, spoon the stew over cooked riced cauliflower.

2 tablespoons all-purpose flour

1 pound beef round, cubed

1 cup sliced carrots

1 cup chopped yellow onion

1 cup sliced celery

1 clove garlic, peeled and finely chopped

¼ teaspoon ground black pepper

¼ teaspoon ground marjoram

¼ teaspoon dried thyme

½ teaspoon salt

2 tablespoons balsamic vinegar

½ cup dry red wine

½ cup water

1 cup sliced button mushrooms

1 Preheat oven to 325°F.
2 Place flour in a large shallow bowl. Dredge beef in flour and place in a 3-quart covered baking dish or Dutch oven. Add carrots, onion, celery, garlic, pepper, marjoram, thyme, salt, and vinegar; combine.
3 Pour red wine and water over mixture. Cover and bake 1 hour.
4 Remove dish from oven. Stir in mushrooms, then return to oven and bake 1 hour, or until beef cubes are tender. Serve.

Southwest Black Bean Burgers

Mixing black beans in with ground beef makes moister, more fla-vorful burgers. And they're lower in fat than the traditional all-beef burger—not to mention higher in fiber.

1 cup cooked black beans

¼ cup chopped yellow onion

1 teaspoon chili powder

1 teaspoon ground cumin

1 tablespoon minced fresh parsley

1 tablespoon minced fresh cilantro

½ teaspoon salt

¾ pound lean ground beef

1 Place beans, onion, chili powder, cumin, parsley, cilantro, and salt in a food processor. Pulse until beans are partially puréed and all ingredients are mixed.

2 In a large bowl, combine ground beef and bean mixture. Shape into 5 patties. Refrigerate covered at least 2 hours.

3 Preheat a gas or charcoal grill to high heat. Brush grill grate with vegetable oil.

4 Grill patties 5 minutes per side. Serve hot.

SERVES 5	
Per Serving:	
Calories	170
Fat	7g
Saturated Fat	3g
Sodium	300mg
Carbohydrates	9g
Fiber	3g
Sugar	1g
Protein	17g

SWAPPING FRESH HERBS FOR DRIED

If you do not have fresh herbs such as parsley or cilantro available, 1 tea-spoon dried can be used in place of 1 tablespoon fresh.

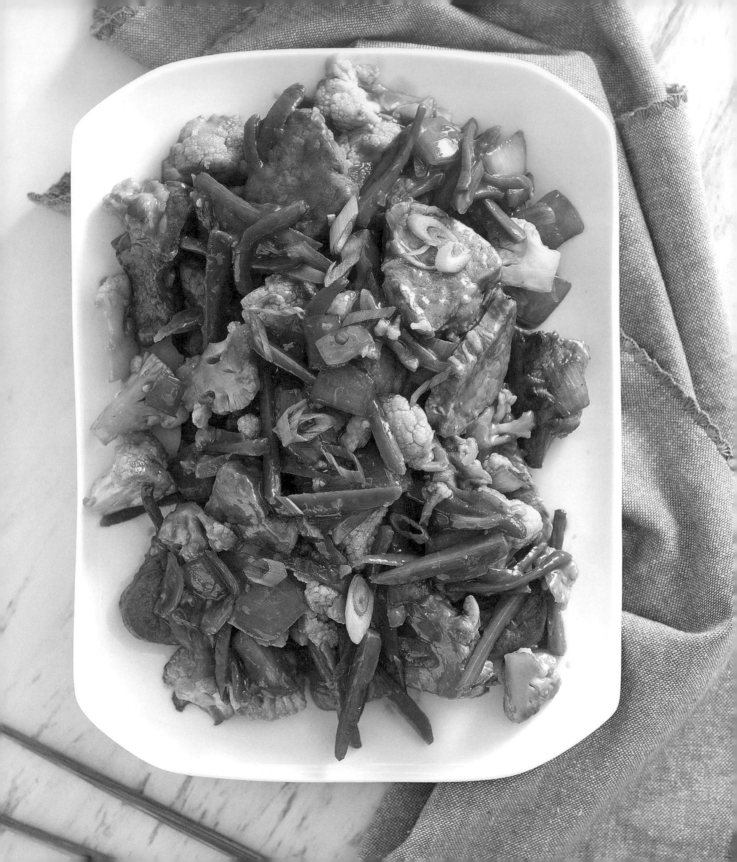

Sweet and Sour Pork Skillet

Homemade sweet and sour sauce glazes this pork and vegetable stir-fry with a terrific flavor—you won't even miss the artificial flavors and excess sugar in the bottled kind.

12 ounces lean pork tenderloin, cut into 1" strips

1 tablespoon amber honey

2 tablespoons rice vinegar

2 teaspoons low-sodium soy sauce

½ teaspoon grated fresh ginger

½ cup chopped yellow onion

½ cup julienne-cut carrots

2 cups cauliflower florets

¼ teaspoon Chinese five-spice powder

2 scallions, sliced

1 In a medium bowl, combine pork, honey, vinegar, soy sauce, and ginger. Toss to coat, then set aside to marinate at least 15 minutes.

2 Heat a large nonstick skillet or wok over high heat 45 seconds. Using a slotted spoon, transfer pork to skillet; reserve marinade. Add onion and stir-fry 3 minutes.

3 Add carrots, cauliflower, and reserved marinade to skillet. Toss together and continue to stir-fry an additional 4 minutes or until vegetables are crisp-tender.

4 Stir in five-spice powder and top with scallions just before serving.

SERVES 4	
Per Serving:	
Calories	130
Fat	2g
Saturated Fat	0.5g
Sodium	160mg
Carbohydrates	8g
Fiber	2g
Sugar	4g
Protein	19g

AROMATIC FIVE-SPICE POWDER

Chinese five-spice powder is a blend of cinnamon, anise, fennel (or star anise), ginger, and clove. Five-spice powder is an essential base seasoning for many Chinese dishes. A little of this aromatic mix goes a long way, giving dishes a hint of sweet, savory, and sour.

Fruited Pork Loin Roast Casserole

SERVES 4

Per Serving:

Calories	230
Fat	2.5g
Saturated Fat	1g
Sodium	100mg
Carbohydrates	44g
Fiber	2g
Sugar	12g
Protein	9g

To enhance the flavor of this dish even more, top it with grated Parmesan cheese and a drizzle of extra-virgin olive oil.

4 small Yukon Gold potatoes, peeled and sliced

2 (2-ounce) pieces trimmed boneless pork loin, pounded flat

1 large red apple, peeled, cored, and sliced

4 dried apricot halves

1 tablespoon chopped red onion

2 tablespoons apple juice

1 Preheat oven to 350°F. Spray a medium baking dish with nonstick cooking spray.

2 Layer half potato slices on bottom of prepared dish; top with 1 piece pork. Arrange apple slices over pork; place apricot halves on top of apple. Sprinkle onion over apricot and apples. Add second piece of pork; layer remaining potatoes atop pork. Drizzle apple juice over casserole.

3 Cover dish and bake 50 minutes until potatoes are tender. Keep casserole covered and let rest 10 minutes after removing from oven before serving.

CHAPTER 12

Seafood

Grilled Chili-Lime Shrimp

SERVES 4

Per Serving:

Calories	45
Fat	0.5g
Saturated Fat	0g
Sodium	320mg
Carbohydrates	1g
Fiber	0g
Sugar	1g
Protein	8g

Made with just four simple ingredients, these flavorful grilled shrimp are delicious served as an appetizer, on top of a salad, in tacos, or with stir-fried vegetables.

¼ cup lime juice
4 teaspoons light brown sugar
½ teaspoon chili powder
8 ounces (about 12–14 pieces) shrimp, peeled and deveined

1 Whisk together lime juice, sugar, and chili powder in a small bowl. Place shrimp in a large zip-top plastic bag and add lime juice mixture. Marinate in refrigerator 2 hours.

2 Preheat a gas or charcoal grill to high heat. Soak four wooden skewers in water 10 minutes.

3 Remove shrimp from bag and discard marinade. Thread 3–4 pieces shrimp on each skewer. Grill 2 minutes per side until shrimp are slightly pink. Serve.

Sesame Shrimp and Asparagus

You can substitute brown rice for the pasta in this dish. To cut the carbohydrates even more, omit the pasta entirely and serve with a salad or steamed greens.

2 teaspoons canola oil

2 cloves garlic, peeled and chopped

1 tablespoon grated fresh ginger

1 pound medium shrimp, peeled and deveined

2 tablespoons dry white wine

½ pound asparagus, woody ends trimmed, cut diagonally into 1" pieces

2 cups cooked whole-grain pasta

½ teaspoon sesame seeds

¼ cup thinly sliced scallions

1 teaspoon sesame oil

1 Heat canola oil in a large wok or nonstick skillet over medium-high heat 30 seconds. Add garlic, ginger, and shrimp and stir-fry until shrimp begin to turn pink, about 2 minutes.

2 Add wine and asparagus to skillet; stir-fry an additional 4 minutes.

3 Add pasta, sesame seeds, scallions, and sesame oil; toss lightly, then remove from heat and serve.

SERVES 4	
Per Serving:	
Calories	230
Fat	5g
Saturated Fat	1g
Sodium	660mg
Carbohydrates	24g
Fiber	1g
Sugar	1g
Protein	21g

WHY DO SHRIMP TURN PINK WHEN THEY ARE COOKED?

Uncooked shrimp have a protein covering that is a grayish color, but once they are heated the protein chains in the covering uncoil, allowing the reddish-orange pigment called *astaxanthin* to be released and change their color.

Grilled Salmon with Roasted Peppers

SERVES 4

Per Serving:

Calories	180
Fat	6g
Saturated Fat	1g
Sodium	105mg
Carbohydrates	6g
Fiber	2g
Sugar	4g
Protein	24g

Sweet and savory ingredients combine nicely to flavor the salmon in this recipe. To save time, purchase jarred roasted peppers, drain them, and slice thinly.

4 (4-ounce) salmon steaks

1 tablespoon low-sodium soy sauce

1 tablespoon light brown sugar

1 tablespoon olive oil

2 large red bell peppers

1 tablespoon balsamic vinegar

½ teaspoon dried thyme

¼ teaspoon ground black pepper

WASABI MARINADE

For an alternate version of this grilled salmon, try a wasabi marinade instead. Wasabi can be purchased in raw form or as a powder or paste. It adds a hot, pungent flavor to fish and works especially well with salmon. To make a marinade, mix 1 teaspoon wasabi powder or paste with 2 tablespoons low-sodium soy sauce, ½ teaspoon grated fresh ginger, and 1 teaspoon sesame oil. Coat fish with the marinade, and marinate covered in refrigerator at least 1 hour before grilling.

1 Place salmon in a large shallow dish.

2 Mix together soy sauce, sugar, and oil in a small bowl; pour marinade over salmon and turn to cover both sides. Marinate covered in refrigerator at least 1 hour.

3 Preheat broiler to high.

4 Place bell peppers on a large ungreased baking sheet or broiler rack and broil about 2" from heat 15 minutes or until skins are blistered and charred. Turn peppers every 5 minutes while broiling.

5 Place cooked peppers in a large bowl and cover with plastic wrap. Set aside 10 minutes.

6 Remove peppers from bowl. Using a sharp paring knife, remove blackened skins. Cut peppers in half, remove seeds, then cut into thin strips. Place in a small bowl and add vinegar, thyme, and black pepper. Stir to combine and set aside.

7 Preheat a gas or charcoal grill to high heat.

8 Remove salmon from marinade and discard marinade. Grill steaks over medium heat 8 minutes. Turn and grill on other side until salmon is cooked and tender, about 4 minutes longer. Remove from heat.

9 Top each salmon steak with marinated roasted red peppers and serve.

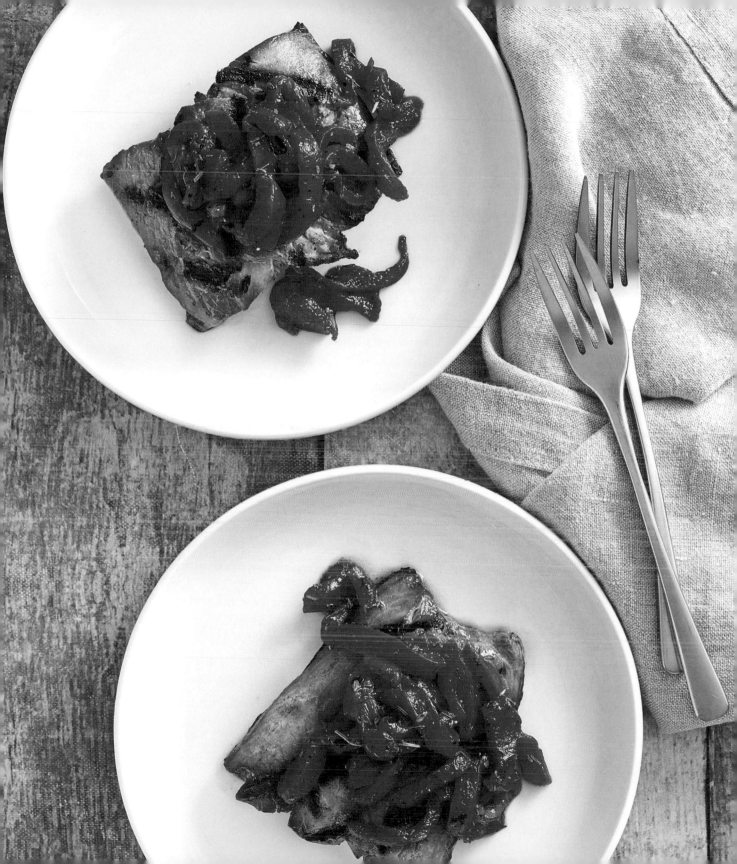

Lemon-Garlic Shrimp and Vegetables

SERVES 2

Per Serving:

Calories	170
Fat	5g
Saturated Fat	1g
Sodium	1,250mg
Carbohydrates	13g
Fiber	2g
Sugar	5g
Protein	20g

Shrimp takes on the flavors of lemon, sesame oil, and honey with a nice mix of nutrient-packed vegetables in this easy stir-fry dish.

2 tablespoons low-sodium soy sauce

1 teaspoon grated lemon zest

1½ tablespoons lemon juice

½ teaspoon amber honey

½ cup water

¼ teaspoon ground black pepper

1 stalk celery, sliced

1 cup shredded red cabbage

½ medium red bell pepper, seeded and thinly sliced

3 cloves garlic, peeled and chopped

½ cup bean sprouts

1 teaspoon sesame oil

½ pound medium shrimp, peeled and deveined

1 In a small bowl, mix together soy sauce, lemon zest, lemon juice, honey, water, and black pepper. Set aside.

2 Spray a large frying pan with nonstick cooking spray and place over medium heat 30 seconds.

3 Add celery and cabbage to pan and sauté 1 minute. Add bell pepper, garlic, and bean sprouts and sauté until all vegetables are crisp-tender, about 5 minutes.

4 Transfer cooked vegetables to a large plate and cover.

5 Add oil to pan used for vegetables, and once oil is hot, about 30 seconds, cook shrimp until opaque, about 2 minutes on each side. Return vegetables to pan with cooked shrimp.

6 Pour soy sauce mixture over shrimp and vegetables and cook 4 minutes until sauce is slightly reduced. Serve.

Slow-Roasted Salmon

Simple ingredients and slow roasting bring out the flavor of this basic but delicious salmon dish. You can serve with lemon wedges or add a dollop of a favorite dressing as an additional garnish.

2 teaspoons extra-virgin olive oil

4 (5-ounce) salmon fillets with skin

1 cup finely minced fresh chives

½ teaspoon sea salt

¼ teaspoon ground white pepper

4 small sprigs sage

SERVES 4	
Per Serving:	
Calories	210
Fat	9g
Saturated Fat	1.5g
Sodium	400mg
Carbohydrates	1g
Fiber	0g
Sugar	0g
Protein	29g

1 Preheat oven to 250°F. Line a large baking sheet with foil and spray with nonstick cooking spray.

2 Rub oil into flesh side of each salmon fillet. Completely cover fillets with chives and gently press them into flesh. Season with salt and pepper on both sides.

3 Place fillets skin-side down on prepared baking sheet. Roast 25 minutes or until flesh flakes easily with a fork.

4 Garnish salmon with sage sprigs and serve.

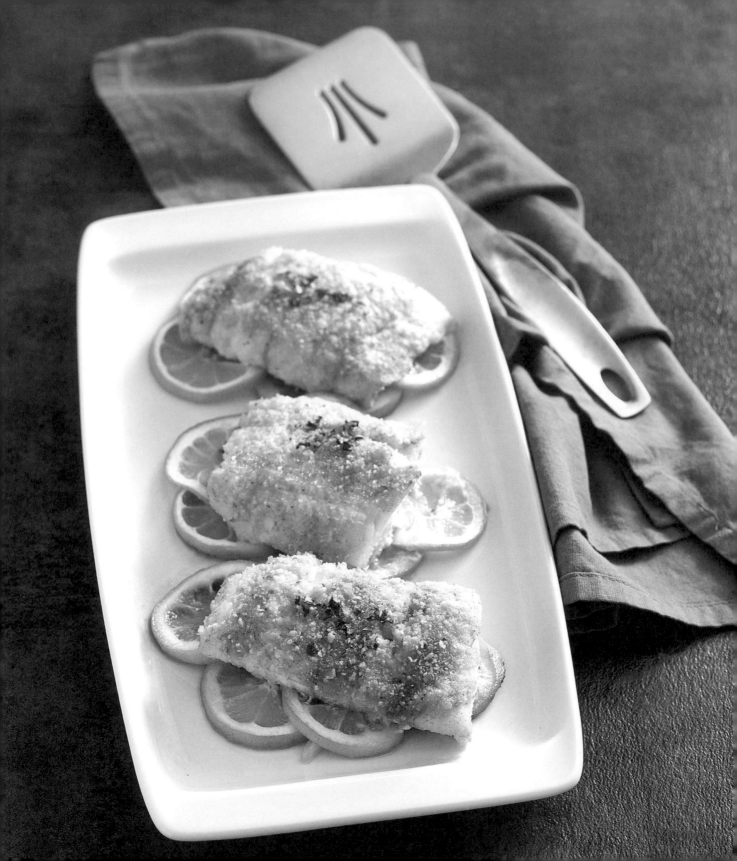

Baked Bread Crumb–Crusted Fish with Lemon

Lemon is the star in this easy-to-make dish. Juice, zest, and lemon slices all add bright, fresh flavor to the mild whitefish.

2 large lemons

¼ cup dried bread crumbs

1½ pounds halibut fillets

½ teaspoon sea salt

¼ teaspoon ground black pepper

1 tablespoon minced fresh parsley

1 Preheat oven to 375°F. Spray a medium baking dish with nonstick cooking spray.

2 Cut 1 lemon into thin slices. Grate 1 tablespoon of zest from second lemon, then squeeze juice into a small bowl.

3 Combine lemon zest and bread crumbs in a separate small bowl; stir to mix.

4 Arrange lemon slices in bottom of prepared baking dish. Dip fish pieces in lemon juice; set on lemon slices.

5 Sprinkle bread crumb mixture evenly over fish, along with salt and pepper. Bake until crumbs are lightly browned and fish is just opaque, about 13 minutes.

6 Transfer fish and lemon slices to a serving dish and sprinkle with parsley. Serve immediately.

SERVES 6

Per Serving:

Calories	130
Fat	2g
Saturated Fat	0g
Sodium	300mg
Carbohydrates	5g
Fiber	1g
Sugar	1g
Protein	22g

LEMON INFUSION

Mildly flavored fish such as catfish, cod, halibut, orange roughy, rockfish, and snapper benefit from the distinctive flavor of lemon. Adding slices of lemon to the dish allows the flavor to infuse into fish.

A-Taste-of-Italy Baked Fish

SERVES 4	
Per Serving:	
Calories	140
Fat	1g
Saturated Fat	0g
Sodium	360mg
Carbohydrates	9g
Fiber	2g
Sugar	5g
Protein	21g

Cod is a mild, low-fat fish that is high in protein. It combines nicely with herbs, onion, and tomatoes. Serve this Mediterranean-style fish with mixed greens or a cooked vegetable for a delicious low-calorie meal.

1 (14.5-ounce) can stewed tomatoes including juice
¼ teaspoon dried minced onion
½ teaspoon dried minced garlic
¼ teaspoon dried basil
¼ teaspoon dried parsley
⅛ teaspoon dried oregano
⅛ teaspoon granulated sugar
1 tablespoon grated Parmesan cheese
1 pound cod fillets

1 Preheat oven to 375°F. Spray a medium baking dish with nonstick cooking spray.
2 Place tomatoes, onion, garlic, basil, parsley, oregano, sugar, and cheese in prepared baking dish and stir to combine.
3 Arrange fillets over tomato mixture, folding thin tail ends under. Spoon some of mixture over fillets. Bake uncovered 22 minutes, or until fish is opaque and flakes easily with a fork. Serve.

Asian-Style Fish Cakes

For a crunchy take on these fish cakes, coat each side in rice flour and then lightly spritz the tops of the patties with olive or peanut oil before baking.

1 (1-pound) catfish fillet, cut into 1" pieces

2 scallions, minced

1 small banana pepper, cored, seeded, and chopped

2 cloves garlic, peeled and minced

1 tablespoon minced fresh ginger

1 tablespoon Bragg Liquid Aminos

1 tablespoon lemon juice

1 teaspoon lemon zest

1 teaspoon Old Bay seasoning

SERVES 8	
Per Serving:	
Calories	70
Fat	3.5g
Saturated Fat	0.5g
Sodium	250mg
Carbohydrates	1g
Fiber	0g
Sugar	0g
Protein	9g

1 Preheat oven to 375°F. Spray a large baking sheet with nonstick cooking spray.

2 Add fish, scallions, banana pepper, garlic, ginger, Braggs Liquid Aminos, lemon juice, and lemon zest in a food processor; process until chopped and mixed.

3 Transfer fish mixture to a large bowl and add Old Bay seasoning; stir to mix. Form mixture into 16 patties.

4 Place patties on prepared baking sheet and bake 13 minutes until crisp. Serve.

Sweet Onion–Baked Yellowtail Snapper

WHAT'S SPECIAL ABOUT SWEET ONIONS

The most common sweet onions are Walla Walla, Maui, and Vidalia. Their sweet flavor is due to a lower amount of sulfur present in the soil they are grown in. They are white or yellow and often have a flatter appearance than regular onions. Sweet onions can be more perishable and should be stored in the refrigerator.

The mild flavor of the snapper pairs nicely with the sweet onions in this quick and easy dish.

2 cups sliced Vidalia onions

1 tablespoon balsamic vinegar

2 teaspoons light brown sugar

4 teaspoons olive oil

1 pound skinless yellowtail snapper fillets

1 In a medium covered microwave-safe dish, microwave onions on high 5 minutes until transparent. Carefully remove cover; stir in vinegar and sugar. Cover and set aside 5 minutes.

2 Heat oil in a medium nonstick skillet over medium-high heat 30 seconds. Transfer steamed onion mixture to skillet and sauté until browned but not crisp, about 2 minutes. Reduce heat to medium and cook until all liquid has evaporated from pan, stirring often, another 3 minutes. Onions should have a shiny and dark caramelized color. (This can be prepared up to 3 days in advance; store tightly covered in refrigerator.)

3 Preheat oven to 375°F. Spray a large baking sheet with nonstick cooking spray.

4 Rinse snapper in cold water and dry between paper towels. Arrange on prepared baking sheet. Spoon caramelized onions over tops of fillets, pressing to form a light crust over top of fish. Bake 13 minutes, or until fish flakes easily with a fork.

5 Serve immediately.

Stir-Fried Ginger Scallops with Vegetables

Fresh ginger combines nicely with these scallops to add wonderful flavor. Serve this dish over brown rice or whole-wheat pasta for a satisfying and healthy dinner.

1 pound sea scallops, rinsed

1 teaspoon peanut oil

1 tablespoon chopped fresh ginger

2 cloves garlic, peeled and minced

4 scallions, thinly sliced

1 teaspoon rice wine vinegar

2 teaspoons low-sodium soy sauce

½ cup low-sodium chicken broth

2 cups broccoli florets

1 teaspoon cornstarch

¼ teaspoon toasted sesame oil

SERVES 4	
Per Serving:	
Calories	140
Fat	2.5g
Saturated Fat	0g
Sodium	280mg
Carbohydrates	7g
Fiber	1g
Sugar	1g
Protein	21g

1 Pat scallops dry between layers of paper towels.

2 Heat peanut oil in a medium deep nonstick skillet or wok about 30 seconds. Add ginger, garlic, and scallions and sauté 2 minutes, being careful ginger doesn't burn. Add vinegar, soy sauce, and broth; bring to a boil, then remove from heat.

3 Put skillet or wok on medium-high heat 30 seconds, then add scallops; sauté 1 minute on each side. (Do scallops in batches if necessary; be careful not to overcook.)

4 Place broccoli in a large, covered microwave-safe dish; pour chicken broth mixture over top. Microwave on high 4 minutes. (Keep in mind that vegetables will continue to steam for a minute or so if cover remains on dish.)

5 Remove scallops and ginger mixture from pan when done; set aside. Drain (but do not discard) liquid from broccoli; transfer broccoli to heated skillet or wok and keep liquid separate in bowl. Stir-fry broccoli to bring up to serving temperature, about 4 minutes.

6 In a small cup or bowl, add a few drops of water to cornstarch to make a slurry.

7 Whisk slurry into reserved broccoli liquid; microwave on high 1 minute. Add sesame oil; whisk again. Pour thickened broth mixture over broccoli; toss to mix. Add scallops back to broccoli mixture; stir-fry over medium heat to return scallops to serving temperature, about 3 minutes.

SLICING SCALLOPS

If a recipe calls for slicing scallops, make sure to avoid cutting them top to bottom or they may fall apart. Slice them horizontally instead.

Crab Cakes with Sesame Crust

SERVING CRAB CAKES

Crab cakes can be served as an appetizer with a squeeze of lemon and a dollop of cocktail sauce. You can also make them into a meal served over mixed greens or with your favorite vegetable soup.

Using sesame seeds instead of bread crumbs gives these crab cakes a unique, delicious flavor and a crispy crust.

¼ **cup lightly toasted sesame seeds**

1 pound lump crabmeat

1 large egg

1 tablespoon minced fresh ginger

1 small scallion, finely chopped

1 tablespoon dry sherry

1 tablespoon lemon juice

6 tablespoons mayonnaise

½ **teaspoon sea salt**

¼ **teaspoon ground white pepper**

¾ **teaspoon Old Bay seasoning**

1 Preheat oven to 375°F. Spray a large baking sheet with nonstick cooking spray. Pour sesame seeds into a medium shallow bowl and set aside.

2 In a separate large bowl, mix together crab, egg, ginger, scallion, sherry, lemon juice, mayonnaise, salt, pepper, and Old Bay seasoning.

3 Form crab mixture into 10 equal cakes. Dip each side of cakes in sesame seeds and arrange cakes on prepared baking sheet.

4 Bake 8 minutes until warmed through and golden brown on each side. Serve immediately.

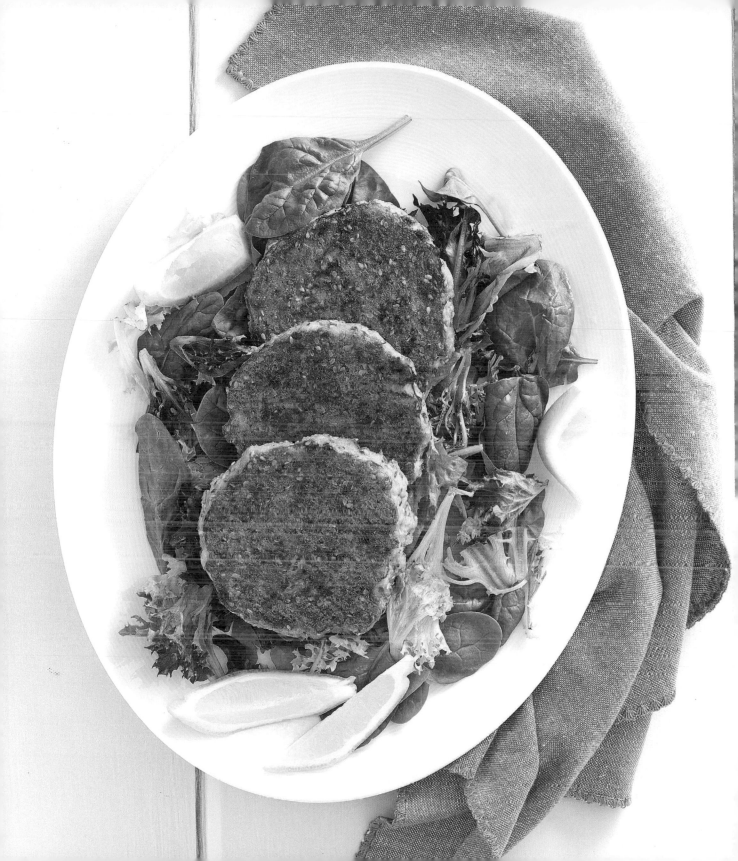

CHAPTER 13

Grains, Pasta, and Potatoes

Brown Rice and Vegetable Sauté

SERVES 4

Per Serving:

Calories	250
Fat	10g
Saturated Fat	1.5g
Sodium	160mg
Carbohydrates	31g
Fiber	3g
Sugar	3g
Protein	15g

BEAN SPROUT NUTRITION

Bean sprouts are low in calories and carbohydrates, and just 1 cup provides 25 percent of the daily requirement for vitamin C. The sprouting process actually increases their antioxidant content quite a bit.

If you are short on time, you can use instant or precooked brown rice to make this vegetarian dish even easier.

1 cup water

½ cup uncooked brown rice

1 tablespoon olive oil

½ cup chopped yellow onion

1 cup chopped red bell pepper

1 teaspoon minced garlic

4 ounces button mushrooms, sliced

1 (12-ounce) package fresh bean sprouts

1 tablespoon low-sodium soy sauce

1 teaspoon grated fresh ginger

1 Place water in a medium saucepan and bring to a boil over high heat. Add rice, reduce heat to low, cover, and simmer 35 minutes until all water is absorbed and rice is tender. Remove from heat and set aside.

2 In a large nonstick skillet or wok, heat oil over medium-high heat 30 seconds. Add onion, bell pepper, and garlic and sauté 7 minutes until onion is translucent.

3 Add mushrooms, bean sprouts, and soy sauce to skillet. Reduce heat to low and cook 3 minutes.

4 Stir in rice and ginger and continue cooking on low 3 minutes. Serve warm.

Squash and Bulgur Pilaf

The nutty, earthy flavor of bulgur combines nicely with the sweet currants, crunchy walnuts, and warm cinnamon of this tasty dish.

1 tablespoon olive oil

½ cup chopped yellow onion

1 teaspoon minced garlic

1½ cups chopped yellow summer squash

1 cup bulgur wheat

2 cups low-sodium chicken broth

½ teaspoon ground cinnamon

¼ cup dried black currants

¼ cup chopped walnuts

1 Heat oil in a large nonstick skillet over medium-high heat 30 seconds. Sauté onion, garlic, squash, and bulgur until onion is tender, about 5 minutes.

2 Stir in broth and cinnamon; heat to boiling. Reduce heat to low and simmer, covered, 10 minutes.

3 Stir in currants and continue to simmer an additional 15 minutes. Stir in walnuts just before serving.

SERVES 6	
Per Serving:	
Calories	190
Fat	7g
Saturated Fat	1.5g
Sodium	45mg
Carbohydrates	27g
Fiber	4g
Sugar	5g
Protein	5g

BENEFITS OF BULGUR

Bulgur is rich in B vitamins, iron, fiber, and protein. It has a nutty, chewy texture and cooks up quickly.

Tabbouleh

SERVES 6

Per Serving:	
Calories	140
Fat	9g
Saturated Fat	1.5g
Sodium	210mg
Carbohydrates	13g
Fiber	3g
Sugar	2g
Protein	2g

Tabbouleh is a classic Mediterranean salad featuring parsley and bulgur wheat. To reduce the carb count per serving, add some steamed riced cauliflower in place of bulgur wheat.

½ cup bulgur wheat

1 cup boiling water

1 cup finely chopped and packed fresh parsley

⅓ cup finely chopped fresh mint

½ cup finely chopped red onion

1 cup chopped cucumber

¼ cup lemon juice

¼ cup olive oil

½ teaspoon salt

¼ teaspoon ground black pepper

1 cup chopped Roma tomato

1 Place bulgur in a small bowl and pour boiling water over it; let stand 20 minutes.

2 Drain bulgur and squeeze out excess water using a colander lined with cheesecloth. Transfer to a medium bowl.

3 Add parsley, mint, onion, and cucumber to bowl. Add lemon juice, oil, salt, and pepper; mix well.

4 Cover and refrigerate at least 3 hours before serving. Just before serving, add tomatoes; toss lightly.

Tuscan Pasta Fagioli

Beans add protein and fiber to this satisfying pasta meal. Top the pasta with chopped fresh basil before serving.

2 tablespoons olive oil

⅓ cup chopped yellow onion

3 cloves garlic, peeled and minced

½ pound Roma tomatoes, peeled and chopped

5 cups low-sodium vegetable stock

¼ teaspoon ground black pepper

3 cups canned cannellini beans, drained and rinsed, divided

2½ cups whole-grain pasta shells

2 tablespoons Parmesan cheese

SERVES 6	
Per Serving:	
Calories	370
Fat	10g
Saturated Fat	2g
Sodium	170mg
Carbohydrates	54g
Fiber	1g
Sugar	6g
Protein	20g

1 Heat oil in a large soup pot or Dutch oven over medium heat 30 seconds. Add onion and garlic and sauté 5 minutes until soft but not browned. Add tomatoes, stock, and pepper.

2 In a food processor or blender, purée 1½ cups beans; add to stock mixture. Cover, reduce heat to medium-low, and simmer 25 minutes, stirring occasionally.

3 Meanwhile, fill a large saucepan ⅔ full with water, cover, and bring to a boil over high heat. Add pasta, return to a boil, and cook uncovered 6 minutes until al dente, then drain.

4 Add pasta and remaining 1½ cups beans to soup pot and simmer 5 minutes. Top with cheese before serving.

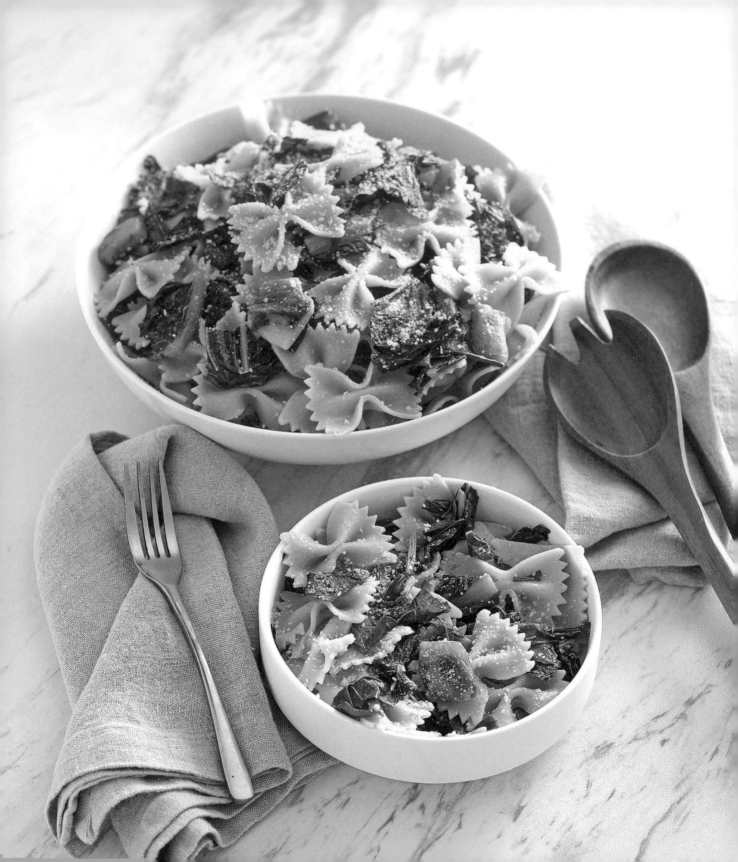

Greens in Garlic with Pasta

Use a light olive oil to sauté the greens—it has a higher smoke point and a neutral taste. The more delicate, fruity extra-virgin olive oil is best used in the dressing.

2 teaspoons light olive oil

4 cloves garlic, peeled and minced

6 cups tightly packed mustard greens

2 cups cooked bow tie pasta

2 teaspoons extra-virgin olive oil

¼ cup freshly grated Parmesan cheese

¼ teaspoon salt

¼ teaspoon ground black pepper

1 Heat light olive oil in a large sauté pan over medium-low heat 30 seconds. Add garlic and sauté 1 minute until golden brown.

2 Add greens; sauté until coated in garlic oil, about 4 minutes. Remove from heat.

3 In a large serving bowl, add pasta, cooked greens, extra-virgin olive oil, cheese, salt, and pepper; toss to mix. Serve immediately.

SERVES 4	
Per Serving:	
Calories	170
Fat	7g
Saturated Fat	1.5g
Sodium	260mg
Carbohydrates	18g
Fiber	0g
Sugar	1g
Protein	6g

SWEET OR SALTY?

In most cases, when you add a pinch (less than ⅛ teaspoon) of sugar to a recipe, you can reduce the amount of salt without noticing a difference. Sugar acts as a flavor enhancer and magnifies the effect of the salt.

Southwestern Pasta Primavera

SERVES 8

Per Serving:

Calories	150
Fat	2g
Saturated Fat	0g
Sodium	230mg
Carbohydrates	28g
Fiber	4g
Sugar	6g
Protein	6g

Garnish this flavorful, vegetable-filled pasta dish with low-fat shredded cheese and chopped cilantro. Serve with grilled chicken or fish for a satisfying meal.

1 teaspoon olive oil

1 cup chopped white onion

1 cup chopped red bell pepper

2 cups chopped zucchini

1 cup canned black beans, drained and rinsed

1 cup corn kernels

1 (14-ounce) can stewed tomatoes including juice

1 tablespoon ground cumin

1 tablespoon chili powder

3 cups cooked whole-wheat pasta

1 Heat oil in a large skillet over medium heat 30 seconds. Add onion and bell pepper and sauté 3 minutes until lightly browned.

2 Add zucchini, beans, corn, tomatoes, cumin, and chili powder to skillet. Simmer 6 minutes, stirring occasionally.

3 Stir in pasta. Cook another 2 minutes until warmed through before serving.

Herbed Quinoa with Sun-Dried Tomatoes

Here's an easy grain-based side to add to chicken or fish and salad for a Mediterranean-inspired meal!

½ tablespoon olive oil

¼ cup chopped yellow onion

1 clove garlic, peeled and minced

1 cup quinoa, rinsed

2 cups low-sodium chicken broth

½ cup sliced button mushrooms

6 sun-dried tomatoes, cut into ¼" pieces

1 teaspoon Italian-blend seasoning

1 Heat oil in a medium saucepan over medium heat 30 seconds. Add onions and garlic and sauté until tender, about 5 minutes, then set aside on a plate.

2 Place quinoa in same saucepan with broth. Bring to a boil over high heat. Boil 2 minutes.

3 Add mushrooms, tomatoes, and Italian seasoning, and cooked onions and garlic to pan. Reduce heat to low and cover. Cook 15 minutes or until all water is absorbed. Serve hot or at room temperature.

SERVES 6

Per Serving:

Calories	130
Fat	3g
Saturated Fat	0g
Sodium	35mg
Carbohydrates	21g
Fiber	2g
Sugar	2g
Protein	5g

COOKING TIME FOR QUINOA

Quinoa takes no longer to cook than rice or pasta, usually about 15 minutes. You can tell quinoa is cooked when grains have turned from white to transparent and spiral-like germ has separated from seed.

Whole-Wheat Couscous Salad

SERVES 8

Per Serving:

Calories	170
Fat	9g
Saturated Fat	1g
Sodium	20mg
Carbohydrates	18g
Fiber	1g
Sugar	5g
Protein	4g

AREN'T CURRANTS JUST SMALL RAISINS?

Dried currants may look like miniature raisins, but they are actually quite different. Currants are berries from a shrub, not a vine, and there are red and black varieties. Black currants are rich in phytonutrients and antioxidants. They have twice the potassium of bananas and four times the vitamin C of oranges!

This grain salad is a tasty side but can also be made into a main meal by adding some cooked beans or chopped chicken.

1 cup low-sodium chicken broth

¼ cup dried black currants

½ teaspoon ground cumin

¾ cup whole-wheat couscous

1 cup chopped broccoli, steamed to crisp-tender

3 tablespoons pine nuts

¼ cup olive oil

2 tablespoons lemon juice

1 tablespoon chopped fresh parsley

1 Combine broth, currants, and cumin in a medium saucepan over high heat and bring to a boil. Remove from heat as soon as it boils and stir in couscous. Cover and set aside 25 minutes until cool. Fluff couscous with a fork three times during cooling process.

2 Add broccoli and pine nuts to cooled couscous.

3 In a small bowl, whisk together oil and lemon juice. Pour over couscous mixture and toss lightly. Garnish with parsley before serving.

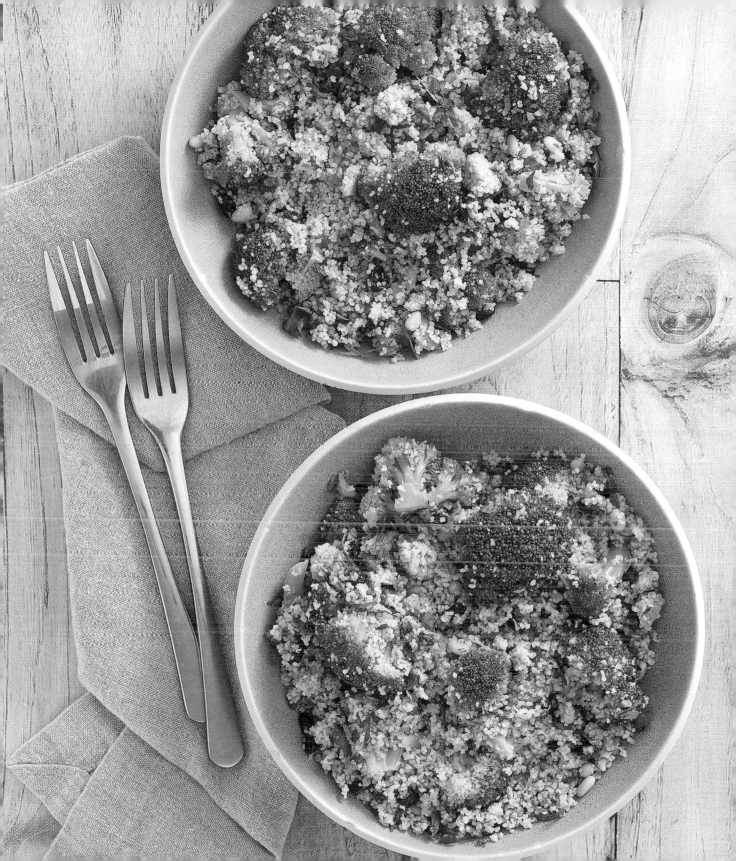

Quinoa with Roasted Vegetables

SERVES 4

Per Serving:

Calories	140
Fat	5g
Saturated Fat	0.5g
Sodium	150mg
Carbohydrates	20g
Fiber	4g
Sugar	4g
Protein	4g

For a spicier version of this dish, replace one of the varieties of bell pepper with a hotter red or green pepper, such as a serrano or jalapeño.

⅔ cup chopped green bell pepper

½ cup chopped red bell pepper

3 cups diced eggplant

2 cloves garlic, peeled and finely chopped

1 tablespoon olive oil

½ teaspoon ground black pepper

¼ teaspoon ground cumin

1 cup water

¼ teaspoon salt

½ cup quinoa, rinsed

1 Preheat oven to 375°F.
2 Combine bell peppers, eggplant, garlic, oil, black pepper, and cumin in an ungreased 2-quart baking dish. Cover and roast 20 minutes.
3 Uncover dish and continue to roast about 30 minutes until vegetables are browned and tender when pierced with a fork. Remove from oven and recover.
4 Bring water and salt to a boil in a medium saucepan over high heat. Add quinoa, bring to a boil, and cook 5 minutes. Cover, remove from heat, and let stand 15 minutes until all water is absorbed into quinoa.
5 Combine roasted vegetables and quinoa in a large bowl and serve.

Oven-Baked Red Potatoes

Lemon juice adds a boost of flavor to these easy potatoes roasted with minimal fat. If you can't find red potatoes, feel free to substitute small yellow ones instead.

1 pound small red potatoes, halved

¼ cup lemon juice

1 teaspoon olive oil

1 teaspoon sea salt

¼ teaspoon ground black pepper

1 Preheat oven to 350°F.

2 Arrange potatoes in a 13" × 9" ovenproof ungreased casserole dish. Combine remaining ingredients in a small bowl and pour over potatoes. Bake about 35 minutes until potatoes are tender, turning four times to baste. Serve.

SERVES 4	
Per Serving:	
Calories	90
Fat	1.5g
Saturated Fat	0g
Sodium	600mg
Carbohydrates	19g
Fiber	2g
Sugar	2g
Protein	2g

REMEMBER THE ROASTING "RACK"

Use caution when roasting potatoes with meat: Potatoes will act like a sponge, soaking up fat. Your best option is to use lean cuts of meat and elevate them and vegetables above fat by putting them on a roasting rack in the pan or making a "bridge" with the celery to elevate the meat. Discard celery when done.

Roasted Garlic Mashed Potatoes

Per Serving:

Calories	120
Fat	2.5g
Saturated Fat	1.5g
Sodium	350mg
Carbohydrates	21g
Fiber	3g
Sugar	3g
Protein	4g

GRAVY SUBSTITUTE

Instead of using gravy, try a sprinkle of crumbled blue cheese or grated Parmesan over mashed potatoes.

Combining steamed cauliflower with mashed potatoes allows you to increase your portion size without significantly changing the flavor of the mashed potatoes.

¾ pound russet potatoes, peeled and quartered

2 cups chopped cauliflower

4 cloves roasted garlic, peeled (see Dry-Roasted Garlic in the Mushroom Caviar recipe in Chapter 7)

1 small yellow onion, peeled and chopped

¼ cup buttermilk

2 tablespoons nonfat cottage cheese

2 teaspoons unsalted butter

½ teaspoon sea salt

¼ teaspoon ground black pepper

1 Fill a medium saucepan ⅔ full with water, cover, and bring to a boil over high heat. Add potatoes and boil uncovered until tender, about 15 minutes. Drain potatoes and transfer to a large mixing bowl.

2 Meanwhile, heat 1" water in a medium saucepan with a steamer insert over high heat until boiling. Reduce heat to low, place cauliflower in steamer, cover, and steam 5 minutes. Remove cauliflower from steamer with a slotted spoon and transfer to bowl with potatoes.

3 Add garlic, onion, buttermilk, cottage cheese, butter, salt, and pepper to bowl. Use an electric beater to whip until fluffy. Serve immediately.

Oat Crepes

These crepes keep well in the refrigerator in a sealed container up to 3 days. Make a batch on the weekend and enjoy a crepe with your favorite filling any day of the week.

½ **cup oat flour**
¼ **cup liquid egg whites**
½ **cup 1% milk**

1 Place flour in a small bowl, form a well in the middle, and pour egg whites into well. Add milk gradually while whisking briskly to form a smooth, thin batter. Let stand 5 minutes.

2 Spray a medium sauté pan generously with nonstick cooking spray and warm over high heat 2 minutes until pan is very hot.

3 Pour ¼ cup batter in a small circle in center of hot pan. Rock and swirl pan in a circular motion while holding it a few inches above heat to get batter to thinly coat pan. Put pan directly on burner.

4 Heat batter about 1 minute until edges start to curl up. Use a large spatula to flip crepe and heat another 45 seconds or so until very lightly browned.

5 Place cooked crepe on a large plate and cover with paper towel. Repeat cooking, spraying pan between each batch, to make 3 more crepes. (The crepes will begin to cook quicker as the pan gets hotter and may take as little as 30 seconds on each side.) Serve.

SERVES 4

Per Serving:

Calories	70
Fat	1.5g
Saturated Fat	0g
Sodium	40mg
Carbohydrates	10g
Fiber	1g
Sugar	2g
Protein	4g

A CREPE FOR ANY OCCASION

Crepes are a versatile base that can house sweet or savory fillings. Fill with cottage cheese and fresh fruit; chicken and tomato sauce; or sautéed spinach, mushrooms, and low-fat cheese for a delicious treat.

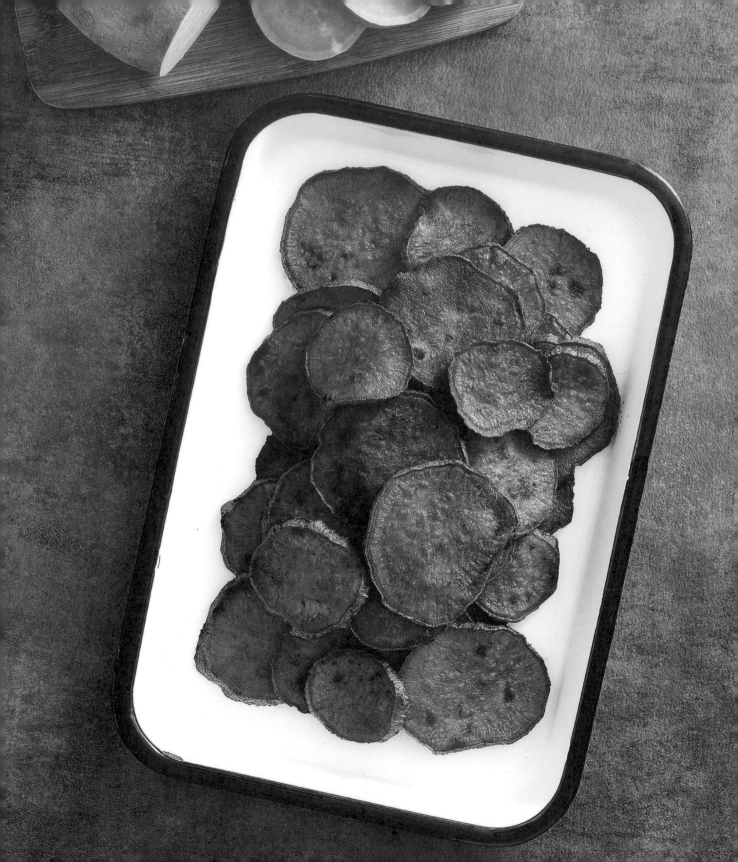

Sweet and Smoky Sweet Potato Slices

Although these hearty potato slices make a good side dish, they're also great for an afternoon snack and taste great either cold or warm.

4 medium sweet potatoes, cut into ⅛" slices (about 5 cups)

2 tablespoons olive oil

2 teaspoons packed light brown sugar

1 tablespoon smoked paprika

½ teaspoon sea salt

1 Preheat oven to 375°F. Spray a large baking sheet with nonstick cooking spray.

2 Place sweet potato slices and oil in a large bowl and toss to coat.

3 In a separate small bowl, combine sugar, paprika, and salt. Sprinkle mixture over sweet potatoes; mix well. Transfer slices to prepared baking sheet.

4 Bake about 25 minutes, flipping once halfway through baking, until lightly browned and slightly crisp.

SERVES 8	
Per Serving:	
Calories	90
Fat	3.5g
Saturated Fat	0g
Sodium	180mg
Carbohydrates	13g
Fiber	2g
Sugar	5g
Protein	1g

THE SMOKED PAPRIKA DIFFERENCE

Smoked paprika is made from dried pimiento peppers that are smoked over an oak fire and then ground into a fine powder. It has a mild, slightly sweet and smoky flavor.

CHAPTER 14

Vegetable Side Dishes

Mexican-Style Cucumber Boats

SERVES 6

Per Serving:

Calories	60
Fat	1g
Saturated Fat	0g
Sodium	120mg
Carbohydrates	9g
Fiber	2g
Sugar	3g
Protein	3g

THE APPEAL OF PERSIAN CUCUMBERS

Persian cucumbers grow to only about 5"–6" long, have thin skins, and are very crunchy and mostly seedless. Low in calories, cucumbers add crunch and fresh taste to salads. For a flavorful snack, sprinkle spears or slices with chili powder or a salt-free seasoning blend.

Scooped-out cucumber halves make a fun (and low-carb) vessel for ingredients commonly used in burritos. Not only are cucumber boats an attractive side dish, but they're also great for party appetizers or afternoon snacks. Two or three of them would even make a quick lunch.

6 tablespoons jarred black bean dip

3 medium Persian cucumbers, halved lengthwise and seeded

2 tablespoons frozen corn kernels, thawed

2 tablespoons finely diced Roma tomato

2 tablespoons chopped black olives

2 tablespoons low-fat shredded Cheddar cheese

Spread 1 tablespoon black bean dip into depression of each cucumber half. Top with 1 teaspoon each corn, tomato, and olives. Sprinkle each cucumber boat with 1 teaspoon cheese and serve immediately.

Honey Lemon Asparagus

Lemon, honey, and asparagus combine for a lovely taste of spring. Use the thinnest spears you can find and make sure you don't over-cook them.

1 tablespoon olive oil

1 pound asparagus spears, woody ends trimmed and cut into 2" pieces

1 tablespoon lemon juice

1 tablespoon amber honey

2 tablespoons chopped walnuts

2 tablespoons golden raisins

SERVES 4	
Per Serving:	
Calories	110
Fat	6g
Saturated Fat	0.5g
Sodium	0mg
Carbohydrates	13g
Fiber	3g
Sugar	10g
Protein	3g

1 Heat oil in a large skillet over medium-high heat 30 seconds. Add asparagus and sauté about 3 minutes until slightly softened.

2 In a small bowl, whisk together lemon juice and honey. Pour mixture over asparagus and stir to coat. Sauté another 1 minute until asparagus is firm but tender when pierced with a fork.

3 Top with walnuts and raisins and serve immediately.

Sesame Snap Peas

SERVES 4

Per Serving:

Calories	80
Fat	4.5g
Saturated Fat	0g
Sodium	0mg
Carbohydrates	6g
Fiber	2g
Sugar	3g
Protein	2g

Both sesame oil and sesame seeds add nutty flavor to this tasty side dish of fresh sweet snap peas. They also make a great snack, cold, straight from the refrigerator.

½ tablespoon canola oil

10 ounces fresh snap peas

¼ cup thinly sliced scallions

1 tablespoon grated fresh ginger

2 teaspoons sesame oil

1 tablespoon sesame seeds

1 Heat canola oil in a large nonstick skillet or wok over medium-high heat 30 seconds. Add snap peas, scallions, and ginger and stir-fry until peas are crisp-tender, about 4 minutes.

2 Stir in sesame oil and sesame seeds; toss lightly and serve.

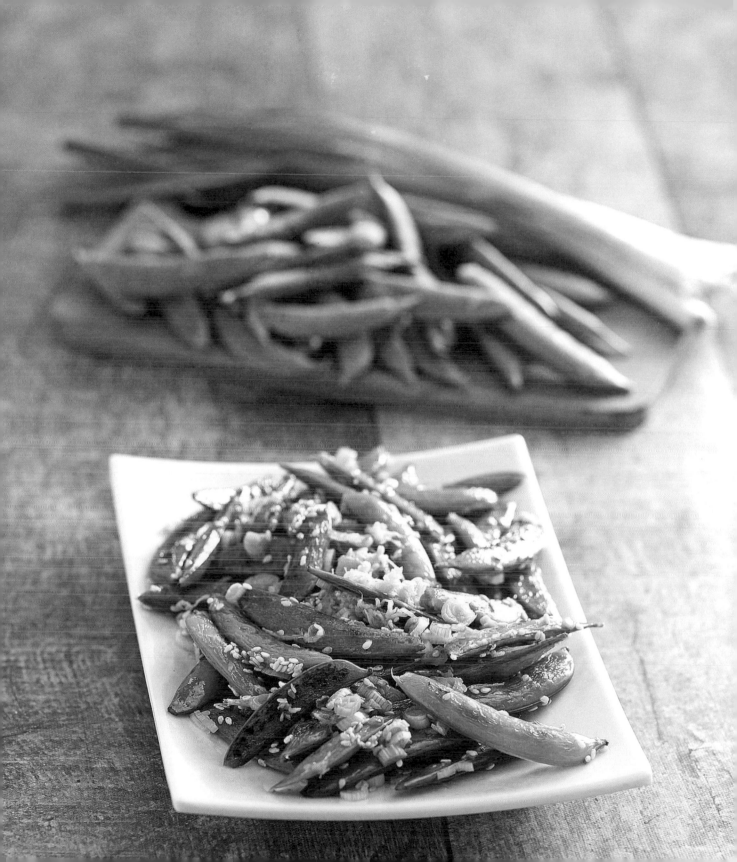

Sautéed Brussels Sprouts with Tomatoes

SERVES 5	
Per Serving:	
Calories	50
Fat	3g
Saturated Fat	0g
Sodium	15mg
Carbohydrates	6g
Fiber	2g
Sugar	2g
Protein	2g

This healthy side dish is easy to make, and the red and green vegetables make it perfect for a holiday dinner.

10 ounces Brussels sprouts, trimmed and halved

1 tablespoon olive oil

¾ cup halved cherry tomatoes

1 Heat 1" water in a medium saucepan with a steamer insert over high heat until boiling. Reduce heat to low and place Brussels sprouts in steamer. Cover and steam 4 minutes.

2 Remove Brussels sprouts from steamer with a slotted spoon and transfer to a large plate lined with paper towels. Pat Brussels sprouts dry with paper towels.

3 Heat oil in a large skillet over medium-high heat 30 seconds. Add Brussels sprouts and sauté 3 minutes until lightly browned.

4 Add tomatoes to skillet and continue to sauté another 1 minute or so until tomatoes have softened. Serve immediately.

Brussels Sprouts Hash with Caramelized Shallots

In a hot oven, Brussels sprouts and shallots caramelize, bringing out their natural sweetness. Serve these alongside eggs or an omelet for a tasty and healthy brunch.

1 pound Brussels sprouts, trimmed and halved

2 medium shallots, peeled and thinly sliced

¼ cup olive oil

½ teaspoon salt

¼ teaspoon ground black pepper

3 tablespoons balsamic vinegar

1 Preheat oven to 400°F.

2 Place Brussels sprouts and shallots in a medium shallow baking dish. Drizzle with oil and season with salt and pepper. Toss to coat.

3 Bake 20 minutes, then remove dish from oven, and drizzle with vinegar. Return dish to oven and bake another 3 minutes. Serve warm.

SERVES 6

Per Serving:

Calories	130
Fat	9g
Saturated Fat	1.5g
Sodium	220mg
Carbohydrates	10g
Fiber	3g
Sugar	4g
Protein	3g

HOW DO SHALLOTS DIFFER FROM ONIONS?

Shallots and onions, along with garlic, are all members of the allium family of vegetables. Shallots are about ⅓ the size of an average onion and are a bit sweeter and milder tasting than onions. They have a hint of garlic flavor as well.

Broccoli Rabe with Pine Nuts

SERVES 4

Per Serving:

Calories	90
Fat	7g
Saturated Fat	0.5g
Sodium	180mg
Carbohydrates	6g
Fiber	3g
Sugar	2g
Protein	4g

PREVENTING BITTER BROCCOLI RABE

Broccoli rabe and other leafy greens (mustard and collard greens) can have a bitter taste once cooked. Rather than add extra salt to offset bitterness, this recipe calls for blanching, which helps reduce bitterness. Blanching should be done as quickly as possible by starting with water at full rolling boil, then removing after 2 minutes of boiling. If allowed to cook too long, the boiling process will reduce the amount of water-soluble nutrients in the vegetables.

Garnish this broccoli rabe with a sprinkle of Parmesan cheese and a squeeze of lemon. This delicious side dish is ready in less than 20 minutes.

¾ **pound broccoli rabe, trimmed and roughly chopped**

1 **tablespoon olive oil**

4 **cloves garlic, peeled and chopped**

¼ **cup chopped sun-dried tomatoes**

2 **tablespoons pine nuts**

¼ **teaspoon salt**

¼ **teaspoon crushed red pepper**

1 Boil 2 quarts water in a large saucepan over high heat. Blanch broccoli rabe in boiling water 2 minutes. Drain well.

2 Heat oil in a large skillet over medium heat 30 seconds; add garlic. Sauté garlic 1 minute, then add blanched broccoli rabe. Toss to coat.

3 Add tomatoes, pine nuts, salt, and crushed red pepper to skillet; cook additional 2 minutes until broccoli rabe is tender, then serve.

French Tarragon Green Beans

Tarragon is added at the end of the cooking to preserve its flavor in this French-inspired dish, combining nicely with fresh green beans.

1½ tablespoons salted butter

¼ cup chopped red onion

1 pound fresh green beans, trimmed

1 tablespoon minced fresh tarragon

1 Melt butter in a medium nonstick skillet over medium heat. Add onion and sauté 5 minutes until translucent.

2 Add green beans to skillet. Cover and steam 2 minutes.

3 Stir in tarragon, cover, and cook an additional 2 minutes. Serve immediately.

SERVES 4	
Per Serving:	
Calories	80
Fat	4.5g
Saturated Fat	3g
Sodium	40mg
Carbohydrates	9g
Fiber	3g
Sugar	4g
Protein	2g

Green Beans in Tomato Sauce

SERVES 10

Per Serving:

Calories	35
Fat	0.5g
Saturated Fat	0g
Sodium	100mg
Carbohydrates	7g
Fiber	2g
Sugar	3g
Protein	1g

Regular green beans are used in this recipe, but you can also try wide Romano green beans. They provide a more robust flavor that pairs well with tomatoes.

4 cups chopped green beans

1 teaspoon olive oil

1 cup chopped yellow onion

2 teaspoons chopped garlic

1 (14.5-ounce) can diced tomatoes including juice

1 teaspoon sweet paprika

1 Place greens beans in a large microwave-safe baking dish with ¼ cup water. Cover and microwave on high 5 minutes, then drain. Set aside.

2 Heat oil in a large skillet over medium-high heat 30 seconds. Add onion and garlic and sauté 3 minutes until lightly browned.

3 Add tomatoes, paprika, and green beans to skillet. Cover, reduce heat to low, and simmer, stirring occasionally, about 10–12 minutes until completely warmed through. Serve.

Simple Sautéed Kale

When doubling this recipe, it is useful to make the batches back-to-back rather than together since the kale takes up a lot of room initially in the pan. Great toppings for this dish include a little salt, pepper, crushed red pepper, garlic powder, or grated Parmesan cheese.

3 teaspoons olive oil, divided

6 packed cups coarsely chopped kale leaves

¼ cup low-sodium vegetable broth

1 Heat 1½ teaspoons oil in a large skillet over medium-high heat 1 minute. Add kale and broth and cook, covered, 5 minutes, stirring occasionally as kale starts to soften.

2 Uncover skillet, stir in remaining 1½ teaspoons oil, mix well, and sauté another 4 minutes before serving.

SERVES 4	
Per Serving:	
Calories	45
Fat	3.5g
Saturated Fat	0g
Sodium	20mg
Carbohydrates	2g
Fiber	1g
Sugar	1g
Protein	1g

WHY IS KALE CONSIDERED A POWER FOOD?

Kale has increased in popularity in the last decade due to it being recognized as one of the more nutrient-dense foods available. At just 30 calories a cup, kale has 3 grams of protein, 2 grams of fiber, and over 100 percent of the daily value for vitamins A, C, and K, as well as decent amounts of some B vitamins, minerals, and other phytochemical antioxidants.

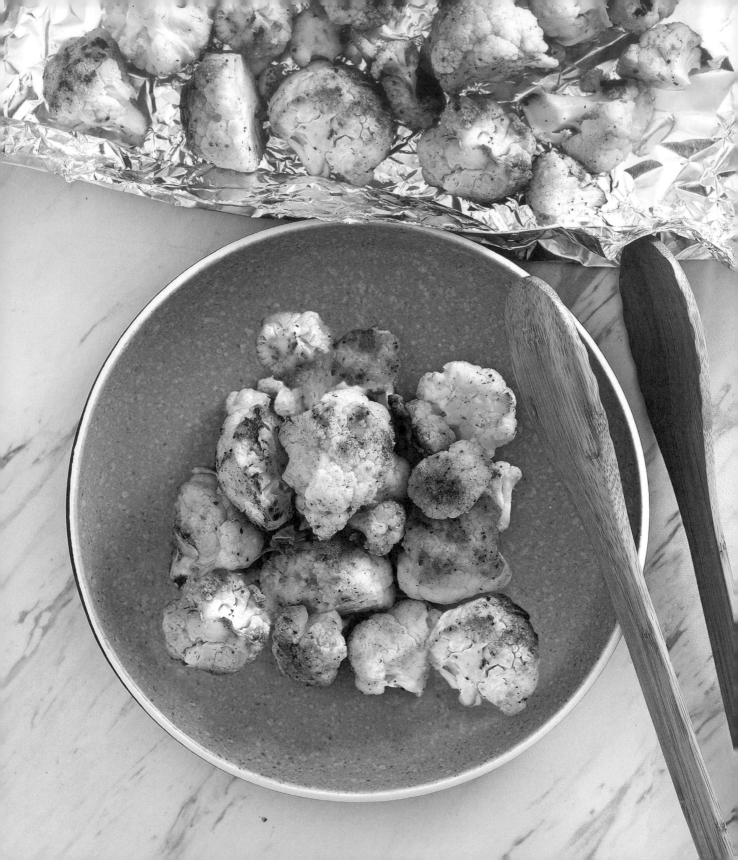

Grilled Cumin Cauliflower

Grilling the cauliflower in foil is an easy way to heat it without worrying about it sticking to or falling though the grill.

3 cups cauliflower florets

1 tablespoon melted salted butter

¼ teaspoon salt

¼ teaspoon ground black pepper

½ teaspoon ground cumin, divided

1 Preheat a gas or charcoal grill to high.

2 Coat a large piece of foil with cooking spray. Put cauliflower in center of foil and drizzle with melted butter. Sprinkle with salt, pepper, and ¼ teaspoon cumin. Fold over sides of foil to make a closed pouch and place on grill.

3 Heat cauliflower 5 minutes, then carefully open foil pouch and turn each piece of cauliflower over.

4 Sprinkle with remaining ¼ teaspoon cumin, close up pouch, and heat another 5 minutes until tender when pierced with a fork. Serve.

SERVES 4	
Per Serving:	
Calories	45
Fat	3g
Saturated Fat	2g
Sodium	170mg
Carbohydrates	4g
Fiber	2g
Sugar	2g
Protein	2g

Honey Mustard–Roasted Carrots and Brussels Sprouts

SERVES 7

Per Serving:

Calories	140
Fat	6g
Saturated Fat	0.5g
Sodium	140mg
Carbohydrates	21g
Fiber	5g
Sugar	13g
Protein	3g

Carrots add a hint of sweetness to Brussels sprouts for this tasty side that works well either hot or cold.

3½ cups quartered Brussels sprouts
3½ cups halved baby carrots
2 tablespoons olive oil, divided
1 tablespoon pure maple syrup
2 tablespoons honey mustard
2 tablespoons finely chopped pecans
2 tablespoons chopped dried cranberries

1 Preheat oven to 350°F. Spray a large baking sheet with nonstick cooking spray.

2 Place Brussels sprouts, carrots, and 1 tablespoon oil in a large bowl and toss to coat.

3 Transfer vegetables to prepared baking sheet and roast 28 minutes, turning them halfway through, until lightly browned and tender when pierced with a fork. Set aside to cool 5 minutes.

4 In a large bowl, whisk together remaining 1 tablespoon oil, maple syrup, and mustard. Add Brussels sprouts mixture, pecans, and cranberries and mix well until evenly coated with dressing. Serve warm or cold.

Zucchini Home Fries

Swap out potatoes for zucchini for a low-carb, low-calorie version of home fries. You'll be pleasantly surprised by how good they taste!

2 teaspoons olive oil, divided

1 medium red bell pepper, seeded and diced

1 medium green bell pepper, seeded and diced

½ cup diced white onion

4 medium zucchini, peeled and diced

½ teaspoon paprika

½ teaspoon chili powder

¼ teaspoon garlic powder

1   Heat 1 teaspoon oil in a large skillet over medium-high heat 30 seconds. Add bell peppers and onion and sauté 4 minutes until crisp-tender.

2   Add remaining 1 teaspoon oil, zucchini, paprika, chili powder, and garlic powder to skillet and sauté another 4 minutes until vegetables are lightly browned and slightly tender. Serve.

SERVES 7	
Per Serving:	
Calories	45
Fat	2g
Saturated Fat	0g
Sodium	20mg
Carbohydrates	7g
Fiber	2g
Sugar	4g
Protein	2g

ADD VEGETABLES TO YOUR BREAKFAST

Pair this recipe with scrambled or poached eggs or fold it into an omelet as an easy way to incorporate vegetables into your morning meal.

Baked Carrot Fries

Baking increases the sweetness of baby carrots. Serve these Baked Carrot Fries as a side dish or a snack with your favorite low-fat dip.

SERVES 8

Per Serving:

Calories	130
Fat	3.5g
Saturated Fat	0g
Sodium	330mg
Carbohydrates	23g
Fiber	6g
Sugar	14g
Protein	3g

6 cups baby carrots

2 tablespoons olive oil

½ teaspoon salt

1 Preheat oven to 400°F. Spray a large baking sheet with nonstick cooking spray.

2 Place carrots and oil in a large bowl and mix well.

3 Spread carrots on prepared baking sheet. Sprinkle with salt and bake 15 minutes. Flip carrots over and bake another 15 minutes until lightly browned and tender when pierced with a fork, then serve.

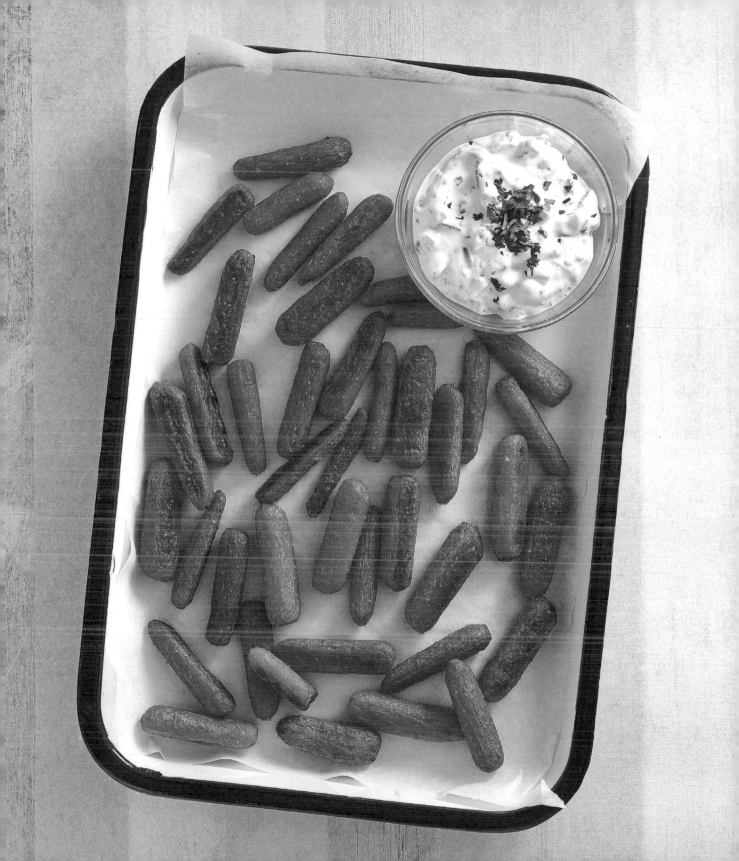

Mashed Cauliflower

Cauliflower works as a satisfying stand-in for potatoes when you're trying to cut calories and carbohydrates. And with all the flavor in this dish you won't miss them.

1 medium head cauliflower

2 tablespoons olive oil

1 tablespoon chopped fresh chives

½ teaspoon salt

½ teaspoon ground black pepper

1 Fill a large pot ⅔ full with water, cover, and bring to a boil over high heat. Add cauliflower and cook uncovered 10 minutes. Drain well, reserving ¼ cup cooking liquid.

2 Place cauliflower in a blender or food processor with oil and reserved cooking liquid. Purée until smooth. Add chives, salt, and pepper and mix before serving.

CHAPTER 15

Desserts and Beverages

Pumpkin Frozen Yogurt Mini Sandwiches

MAKES 16 MINI SANDWICHES

Per Serving (1 sandwich):

Calories	170
Fat	9g
Saturated Fat	1g
Sodium	35mg
Carbohydrates	14g
Fiber	1g
Sugar	7g
Protein	9g

PUMPKIN PURÉE VERSUS PUMPKIN PIE FILLING

Cans of pumpkin purée and pumpkin pie filling are often stacked next to each other in grocery store aisles, but there are some key differences. Pumpkin purée contains only pumpkin and sometimes salt. Pumpkin pie filling contains many more ingredients, including cinnamon, ginger, cloves, allspice, nutmeg, and sugar.

These mini treats, packed with whole grains, healthy fat, and a good amount of protein, will satisfy a sweet craving for dessert. They can even be eaten for breakfast!

12 ounces nonfat vanilla Greek yogurt

1 cup creamy unsalted natural almond butter

⅓ cup pure maple syrup

3 tablespoons pumpkin purée

2 teaspoons light brown sugar

1 teaspoon vanilla extract

¼ teaspoon pumpkin pie spice

⅛ teaspoon salt

¾ cup unflavored protein powder

½ cup old-fashioned rolled oats

1 Place yogurt in a medium bowl, cover, and freeze 1 hour.
2 Meanwhile, combine almond butter, maple syrup, pumpkin purée, sugar, vanilla, pumpkin pie spice, and salt in a separate medium bowl and mix well. Stir in protein powder and oats.
3 Divide dough mixture in half. On a large sheet of parchment paper, form each half into an 8" square.
4 Spread partially frozen yogurt over one square and top with second square. Wrap in parchment paper or foil and freeze 5 hours.
5 Remove from freezer and cut into sixteen squares. Serve cold. Wrap any leftovers in foil or parchment and store in the freezer for up to 3 months.

Almond Cookies

These cookies are not too sweet, with a nutty taste and crunchy texture. Try them with a hot cup of tea.

2 cups roasted unsalted almonds, chopped, divided

¼ cup pecan halves, chopped

½ teaspoon salt

⅓ cup old-fashioned rolled oats

⅓ cup ground flaxseed

1 teaspoon baking powder

1 teaspoon vanilla extract

1 teaspoon ground cinnamon

3 tablespoons unsalted butter, softened

⅔ cup amber honey

MAKES 36 COOKIES	
Per Serving:	
Calories	80
Fat	6g
Saturated Fat	1g
Sodium	30mg
Carbohydrates	8g
Fiber	1g
Sugar	5g
Protein	2g

1 Preheat oven to 350°F. Line a large baking sheet with parchment paper.

2 Set aside 3 tablespoons chopped almonds, then spread pecans and remaining almonds on prepared baking sheet. Bake 7 minutes until lightly toasted. Leave oven on and set aside parchment-lined baking sheet.

3 Place nuts in a food processor and grind until a butter-like consistency forms. Add salt, oats, flaxseed, baking powder, vanilla, cinnamon, and butter. Pulse a few times to combine. Add honey and process until incorporated.

4 Form dough into 1" balls and place on prepared baking sheet; flatten balls slightly. Sprinkle with reserved chopped almonds.

5 Bake 10 minutes until just slightly browned. Cool 15 minutes, then serve. Store leftovers in an airtight container in the refrigerator for up to 1 week.

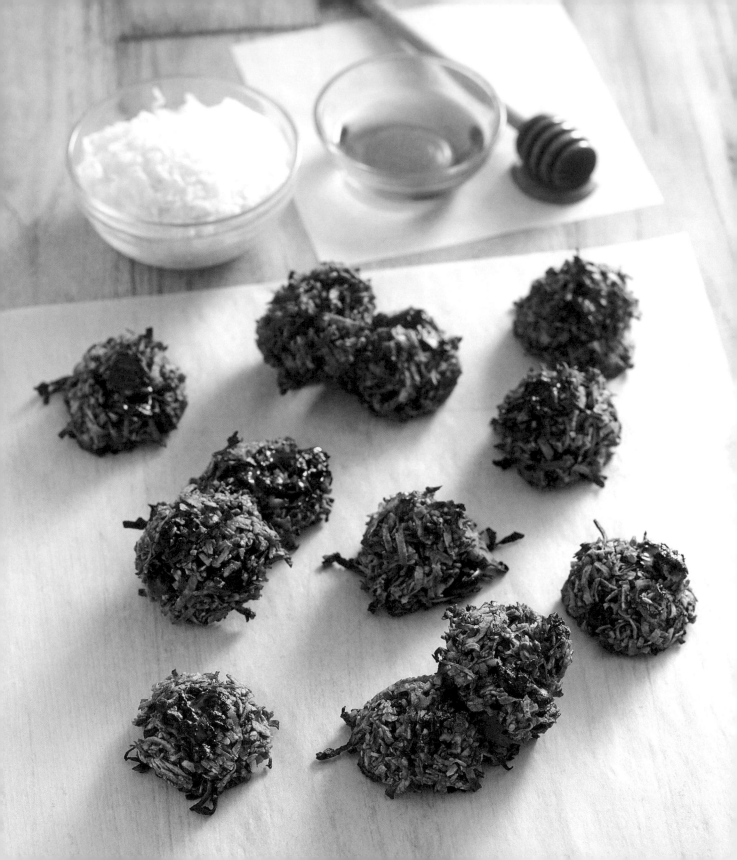

Double Chocolate Macaroons

These macaroons are rich in chocolate flavor. They are also reasonably low in sugar, carbohydrates, and calories.

2 tablespoons oat flour

1¼ cups unsweetened shredded coconut

2 teaspoons cocoa powder

¼ cup amber honey

¼ cup liquid egg whites

2 tablespoons mini chocolate chips (used baking chips, semisweet chocolate)

1 Preheat oven to 350°F. Grease a large baking sheet with nonstick cooking spray.

2 Combine flour, coconut, and cocoa powder in a small bowl. In a separate large bowl, beat together honey and egg whites.

3 Slowly add flour mixture to egg white mixture and stir until thoroughly mixed. Fold in chocolate chips.

4 Drop teaspoonfuls of batter onto prepared baking sheet and bake 16 minutes until tops are firm and cookies are very lightly browned.

5 Transfer cookies to a cooling rack and cool completely, about 15 minutes, before serving.

MAKES 15 MACAROONS

Per Serving (1 macaroon):

Calories	80
Fat	5g
Saturated Fat	4.5g
Sodium	10mg
Carbohydrates	8g
Fiber	1g
Sugar	5g
Protein	1g

MAKE YOUR OWN OAT FLOUR

You can easily make oat flour at home by processing a few cups of old-fashioned oats in a blender or food processor. Blend until a fine powder is formed. Use a sifter to separate out any larger bits.

Brownie Bites

SERVES 16

Per Serving:

Calories	100
Fat	6g
Saturated Fat	1.5g
Sodium	20mg
Carbohydrates	9g
Fiber	1g
Sugar	5g
Protein	2g

This no-bake dessert is really easy to make, fairly low in carbohydrates and sugar, and delicious too. They're great with a cup of coffee or glass of nonfat milk.

½ cup creamy unsalted natural almond butter

3 tablespoons amber honey

1½ tablespoons cocoa powder

⅛ teaspoon salt

½ cup old-fashioned rolled oats

¼ cup semisweet chocolate chips, finely chopped

3 tablespoons whipped cream cheese

4 strawberries, hulled and quartered

PARCHMENT PAPER

Parchment is a heat-resistant, nonstick paper that has a variety of uses in cooking and baking. It can line baking sheets and cake pans to prevent sticking and decrease browning. It can also be helpful for pouring ingredients, making pouches to steam fish, meats, and vegetables, or providing a clean surface to roll out dough. Waxed paper can't be heated because the wax lining will melt.

1 Line an 8" square baking pan with parchment paper.
2 In a medium bowl, combine butter, honey, cocoa, and salt and mix well. Stir in oats and chopped chocolate.
3 Press mixture into prepared pan. Refrigerate 1 hour or freeze 15 minutes.
4 Cut into sixteen squares. Roll each square into a ball and place on a second sheet of parchment paper. Top each ball with ½ teaspoon cream cheese and 1 strawberry quarter before serving. Store leftovers in an airtight container in the refrigerator for up to 1 week.

Seedy Oat Bark

Packed with nutritious grains and seeds, this slightly sweet bark makes a great snack. Try it crumbled over plain Greek yogurt. Quinoa provides protein and a crunchy texture.

½ cup cooked white quinoa

½ cup raw pepitas

½ cup old-fashioned rolled oats

¼ cup chia seeds

1 tablespoon granulated sugar

2 tablespoons melted coconut oil

¼ cup pure maple syrup

1 Preheat oven to 325°F and line a large baking sheet with parchment paper.

2 In a large mixing bowl, combine all ingredients.

3 Pour mixture onto prepared baking sheet and use a metal spoon to spread evenly across pan. It should be thin but solid, with none of pan showing through bark.

4 Bake 15 minutes, then rotate pan and bake an additional 5 minutes or so until lightly browned. Remove from oven and let cool completely, about 15 minutes.

5 Break bark into nine pieces. Serve immediately or store in an airtight container at room temperature up to 1 week.

SERVES 9	
Per Serving:	
Calories	160
Fat	9g
Saturated Fat	3.5g
Sodium	35mg
Carbohydrates	17g
Fiber	4g
Sugar	7g
Protein	4g

SWEET AND SAVORY QUINOA

Cooked quinoa is great as a savory side dish with all kinds of seasonings. Many people don't know that it is also great when mixed with fruit for a fruit salad, used in baking, or as a breakfast cereal. There are many types of quinoa, but the most common are red, white, and a combination of the two. For sweet recipes, the mildly flavored white variety is preferred.

Fall Fruit with Yogurt Sauce

SERVES 8

Per Serving:

Calories	80
Fat	3g
Saturated Fat	0g
Sodium	20mg
Carbohydrates	18g
Fiber	2g
Sugar	15g
Protein	2g

Fall fruit favorites are topped with a lightly sweetened yogurt sauce for a tasty and healthy treat, as a nice breakfast side or delicious dessert.

2 cups chopped red apple

1½ cups halved red seedless grapes

1½ cups chopped pears

2 teaspoons lemon juice, divided

1 cup low-fat vanilla yogurt

1 tablespoon amber honey

¼ cup chopped walnuts

1 Combine apples, grapes, and pears in a medium bowl. Drizzle 1 teaspoon lemon juice over fruit.

2 In a separate small bowl, combine yogurt, remaining 1 teaspoon lemon juice, and honey.

3 Spoon yogurt dressing over fruit and top with walnuts before serving. Store extra fruit and yogurt sauce in separate airtight containers in the refrigerator for up to 2 days.

Bananas Foster

Sweet bananas combine with cool, creamy frozen yogurt for a light and healthy treat. Warming bananas takes their flavor to a whole new level.

4 large ripe bananas, peeled and sliced into ½"-thick slices

¼ cup apple juice concentrate

1 tablespoon grated orange zest

¼ cup pulp-free orange juice

1 tablespoon ground cinnamon

12 ounces nonfat frozen vanilla yogurt

1 Combine bananas, apple juice concentrate, zest, orange juice, and cinnamon in a large nonstick skillet. Bring to a boil over medium-high heat and cook, stirring, 5 minutes until bananas are tender.

2 Scoop 3 ounces frozen yogurt into each of four dessert bowls or stemmed glasses; spoon banana sauce over tops and serve immediately.

SERVES 4

Per Serving:

Calories	250
Fat	0g
Saturated Fat	0g
Sodium	80mg
Carbohydrates	60g
Fiber	5g
Sugar	33g
Protein	6g

KNOW YOUR INGREDIENTS

Overripe bananas are higher in sugar and can adversely affect blood glucose levels. Freeze bananas in skins until ready to use. Doing so makes them perfect additions for fruit smoothies or fruit cups. Remove from freezer and run a little water over peel to remove any frost. Peel using a paring knife and slice according to recipe directions. Frozen bananas can be added directly to smoothies and other recipes.

Strawberry Almond Tarts

SERVES 16

Per Serving:

Calories	100
Fat	6g
Saturated Fat	1g
Sodium	15mg
Carbohydrates	12g
Fiber	1g
Sugar	6g
Protein	2g

SERVING TIP

These tarts will start to get very soft if left out for more than 10 minutes, so they are best served while they are frozen or only slightly thawed.

Whole grains and fresh fruit combine nicely in these bite-sized beauties. They are sure to be a crowd-pleaser at your next party.

½ cup creamy unsalted creamy natural almond butter

¼ cup plus 1 tablespoon amber honey, divided

¾ cup old-fashioned rolled oats

2 tablespoons oat flour

¾ cup hulled and sliced fresh strawberries

⅓ cup light cream cheese

1 tablespoon lemon juice

8 large strawberries, hulled and halved

1 Mix butter, ¼ cup honey, oats, and flour in a medium bowl. Roll mixture out into an 8" × 8" square and cut it into sixteen equal pieces. Roll each piece into a ball and place in cups of a mini-muffin tin. Press dough against bottoms and sides of tin cups to form crusts.

2 Place sliced strawberries, cream cheese, remaining 1 tablespoon honey, and lemon juice in a medium bowl and beat with an electric mixer until blended together and strawberries are mostly puréed. (There will be small bits of berries.)

3 Spoon filling over crusts, dividing evenly. Top each tart with a strawberry half. Freeze 4 hours until centers are very firm. Serve frozen. Store leftovers in an airtight container in the freezer for up to 2 weeks.

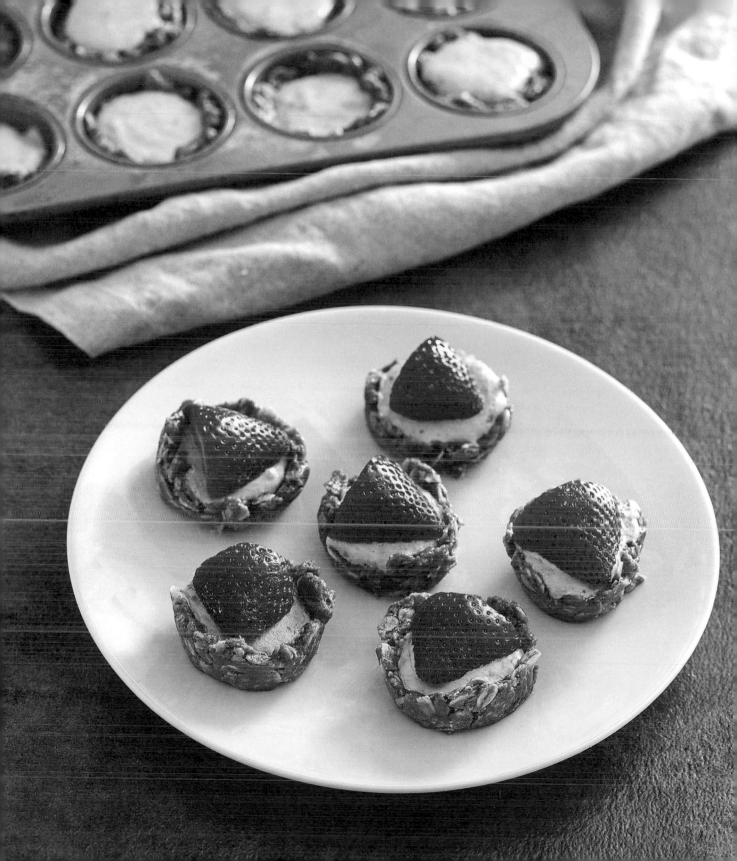

Glazed Carrot Cake

SERVES 9

Per Serving:

Calories	150
Fat	1.5g
Saturated Fat	0g
Sodium	170mg
Carbohydrates	30g
Fiber	2g
Sugar	12g
Protein	4g

This lightened-up version of a classic cake replaces the typical fat-laden cream cheese frosting with a light apple glaze.

1½ cups all-purpose flour

1 teaspoon baking powder

1 teaspoon baking soda

1½ teaspoons ground cinnamon

¼ teaspoon ground cloves

¼ teaspoon ground allspice

⅛ teaspoon ground nutmeg

1 tablespoon granulated sugar

4 tablespoons frozen unsweetened apple juice concentrate, divided

2 large eggs

2 tablespoons ground flaxseed

¼ cup plus 1 tablespoon water, divided

1 teaspoon vanilla extract

3 tablespoons nonfat plain yogurt

1 cup canned unsweetened crushed pineapple, ¼ cup juice retained

1 cup finely shredded carrots

¼ cup raisins

1 Preheat oven to 350°F. Spray an 8" baking pan with nonstick cooking spray.

2 Sift flour, baking powder, baking soda, cinnamon, cloves, allspice, and nutmeg into a large bowl.

3 Place sugar, 2 tablespoons apple juice concentrate, and eggs in a separate large bowl and beat until well mixed.

4 Stir flaxseed and ¼ cup water in a small microwave-safe bowl; microwave on high 30 seconds, then stir. (Mixture should be the consistency of egg whites; if not, microwave at 15-second increments until it is.)

5 Add flaxseed mixture, vanilla, yogurt, and ¼ cup pineapple liquid to egg mixture and mix well.

6 Stir in flour mixture and beat until incorporated. Fold in pineapple, carrots, and raisins.

7 Spoon mixture into prepared pan and bake 22 minutes.

8 Remove from oven and allow cake to cool while you prepare glaze.

9 Mix remaining 2 tablespoons apple juice concentrate with 1 tablespoon water in a small bowl until melted. Spread evenly over cake.

10 Serve warm or at room temperature. Store leftovers in an airtight container in the refrigerator for up to 3 days.

Baked Apples

Warm fruit- and nut-filled apples serve as a healthy substitute for apple pie. You won't miss the crust!

4 large red apples

1 tablespoon light brown sugar

1 teaspoon ground cinnamon

1 tablespoon pure maple syrup

1 tablespoon plus ⅔ cup water, divided

2 tablespoons chopped pecans

2 tablespoons dried cranberries

1 teaspoon light margarine

SERVES 8	
Per Serving:	
Calories	110
Fat	2g
Saturated Fat	0g
Sodium	5mg
Carbohydrates	24g
Fiber	3g
Sugar	18g
Protein	1g

1 Preheat oven to 350°F.

2 Core apples, stopping short ½" from bottoms. Place apples in a shallow 2-quart baking dish.

3 In a small bowl, mix sugar and cinnamon together and whisk in syrup and 1 tablespoon water. Stir in pecans and cranberries. Spoon mixture into apple centers.

4 Top each apple with ¼ teaspoon margarine.

5 Add remaining ⅔ cup water to bottom of dish and cover dish with a lid or foil. Bake about 40 minutes until apples are soft when pierced with a fork or toothpick. Serve warm. Store leftovers in an airtight container in the refrigerator for up to 3 days.

Apple Ginger Super Smoothie

SERVES 2

Per Serving:

Calories	140
Fat	1g
Saturated Fat	0g
Sodium	100mg
Carbohydrates	21g
Fiber	5g
Sugar	12g
Protein	15g

VEGETABLES IN A SMOOTHIE

Spinach adds lots of color but little flavor to a well-balanced smoothie. Fresh spinach can be substituted for the frozen, with 2 cups fresh equal to 1 cup frozen. Frozen ingredients keep the smoothie extra cold, and no ice is needed during blending. The addition of ginger can mask the flavor of any other vegetables you may want to throw in, like carrot, cucumber, or celery.

When it's hot outside, nothing beats a smoothie for breakfast or lunch. Using nonfat plain Greek yogurt provides a satisfying amount of protein. With the addition of spinach, this smoothie helps meet your daily vegetable intake goals as well.

1 cup nonfat plain Greek yogurt

1 small green apple, cored and sliced

¼ cup frozen pineapple

1 cup frozen spinach

1 teaspoon minced fresh ginger

⅛ teaspoon ground cinnamon

Combine all ingredients in a blender and process until smooth. Add water if consistency is too thick.

Kicked-Up Turmeric Lemonade

Turmeric contains curcumin, which can help inflammation and keep blood sugar levels steady. Plus, it gives this lemonade a beautiful golden hue.

2 cups water

¼ cup lemon juice

2 teaspoons amber honey

¼ teaspoon ground turmeric

⅛ teaspoon ground ginger

⅛ teaspoon cayenne pepper

1 Heat water in a small saucepan over high heat to almost boiling, about 5 minutes. Stir in honey until it dissolves, then remove from heat.

2 Add lemon juice, turmeric, ginger, and cayenne to pan and mix well. Refrigerate covered at least 2 hours before serving. Store leftovers in an airtight container in the refrigerator for up to 2 days.

SERVES 2	
Per Serving:	
Calories	30
Fat	0g
Saturated Fat	0g
Sodium	10mg
Carbohydrates	8g
Fiber	0g
Sugar	6g
Protein	0g

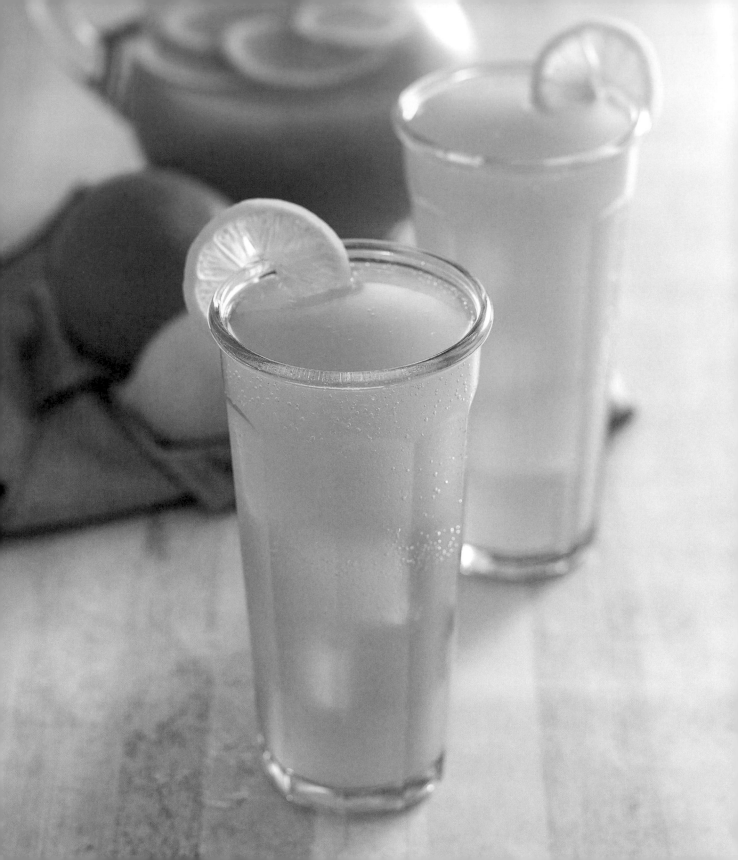

Sparkling Fruited Iced Tea

Serve this delicious and refreshing tea at parties for a healthier-than-soda option. The combination of green tea and fruit is sure to be a crowd-pleaser.

6 cups brewed caffeine-free green tea

2 cups pulp-free orange juice

3 tablespoons lemon juice

16 ounces ginger ale

4 cups seltzer

1 small orange, thinly sliced

1 small lemon, thinly sliced

1 In a large pitcher or punch bowl, mix together tea, orange juice, and lemon juice. Slowly stir in ginger ale and seltzer.

2 Add orange and lemon slices. Serve over ice in tall glass. Store leftovers in an airtight container in the refrigerator for up to 1 day.

SERVES 8

Per Serving:

Calories	60
Fat	0g
Saturated Fat	0g
Sodium	5mg
Carbohydrates	14g
Fiber	1g
Sugar	12g
Protein	1g

GREEN TEA AND DIABETES

A 2006 study by Hiroyasu Iso and others of the JACC Study Group in Japan found that people who drank 6 or more cups of green tea a day were one-third less likely to develop type 2 diabetes than people who drank less than 1 cup of green tea each week. A Taiwanese study from 2003 found that people who drank green tea regularly for more than a decade had smaller waists and a lower body fat composition than those who weren't regular consumers of green tea.

Frothy Orange Jewel

SERVES 1

Per Serving:

Calories	130
Fat	0g
Saturated Fat	0g
Sodium	130mg
Carbohydrates	22g
Fiber	0g
Sugar	9g
Protein	9g

If you don't have fresh orange juice on hand for this recipe, you can substitute 1 tablespoon of frozen orange juice concentrate and 3 tablespoons of water.

¼ **cup pulp-free orange juice**

1 cup skim milk

1½ teaspoons confectioners' sugar

½ **teaspoon vanilla extract**

2 ice cubes

Combine all ingredients in a blender; process until mixed. Serve in a tall glass.

A 2-Week Sample Meal Plan

Use this 2-week plan to help with shopping and prep so you can be ready with fresh, nutritious meals and snacks. It includes some snack options from the recipes in this book, along with the recommendation to have a serving of fresh fruit and/or 1 cup of a vegetable as a snack every day. Note: A fruit serving can be 1 small whole fruit such as an apple, orange, or pear; 1 cup of strawberries; $3/4$ cup blueberries; 10 cherries; 2 clementines; 1 cup cubed melon; or 17 grapes. Good raw non-starchy vegetable snack choices include celery sticks, bell pepper slices, carrot sticks, cucumber slices, mushrooms, and cherry tomatoes.

This plan also includes the option to eat two meals out each week. (Keeping to no more than two meals out will help you stay on track and limit added calories, fat, and sodium.) In addition, it involves using leftovers from recipes to decrease the amount of preparation and minimize food waste.

Week 1

	Breakfast	Lunch	Snack	Dinner
Day 1	2 Banana Walnut Protein Muffins (Chapter 6)	Honey-Dijon Tuna Salad (Chapter 8)	2 tablespoons Italian-Style Bean Dip (Chapter 7) with 1 cup raw vegetables, and one serving of fruit	Vegetable and Bean Chili (Chapter 9) with Crunchy Radish and Celery Salad (Chapter 8)
Day 2	Super Greens Crustless Quiche (Chapter 6)	Vegetable and Bean Chili (Chapter 9) with Crunchy Radish and Celery Salad (Chapter 8)	Banana Walnut Protein Muffins (Chapter 6) and one serving of fruit	Honey and Cider–Glazed Chicken (Chapter 11) with Vegetable Pot Stickers (Chapter 10)
Day 3	Quinoa Berry Breakfast (Chapter 6)	Super Greens Crustless Quiche (Chapter 6)	2 tablespoons Italian-Style Bean Dip (Chapter 7) with 1 cup raw vegetables, and one serving of fruit	Slow Cooker Taco Soup (Chapter 9)
Day 4	Bacon and Egg Breakfast Fried Rice (Chapter 6)	Slow Cooker Taco Soup (Chapter 9)	Snack Mix (Chapter 7) and one serving of fruit	Baked Broccoli and Tofu (Chapter 10) with Vegetable Pot Stickers (Chapter 10)
Day 5	Apple Ginger Super Smoothie (Chapter 15)	Bacon and Egg Breakfast Fried Rice (Chapter 6)	Snack Mix (Chapter 7) and one serving of fruit	Dinner out
Day 6	Buckwheat Pancakes (Chapter 6)	Portobello Mexican Pizzas (Chapter 10)	Bananas Foster (Chapter 15)	Spicy Turkey Burgers (Chapter 11) with Napa Cabbage Slaw (Chapter 8)
Day 7	Tomato and Basil Baked Egg Cups (Chapter 6)	Lunch out	One serving of fruit and 10 almonds	Herbed Chicken and Brown Rice (Chapter 11) with French Tarragon Green Beans (Chapter 14)

Week 2

	Breakfast	Lunch	Snack	Dinner
Day 1	Tomato and Basil Baked Egg Cups (Chapter 6)	Herbed Chicken and Brown Rice (Chapter 11) with French Tarragon Green Beans (Chapter 14)	Seedy Oat Bark (Chapter 15) and one serving of fruit	Broccoli and Whole-Grain Pasta Soup (Chapter 9)
Day 2	2 Carrot Zucchini Spice Muffins (Chapter 6)	Broccoli and Whole Grain Pasta Soup (Chapter 9)	Seedy Oat Bark (Chapter 15) and one serving of fruit	Lemon-Garlic Shrimp and Vegetables (Chapter 12)
Day 3	Buckwheat Pancakes (Chapter 6)	Chipotle Chicken Wraps (Chapter 11)	Honey Raisin Bar (Chapter 7) and one serving of fruit	Southwestern Pasta Primavera (Chapter 13)
Day 4	2 Carrot Zucchini Spice Muffins (Chapter 6)	Southwestern Pasta Primavera (Chapter 13)	Honey Raisin Bar (Chapter 7) and one serving of fruit	Slow-Roasted Salmon (Chapter 12) with Sesame Snap Peas (Chapter 14)
Day 5	Vegetable Frittata (Chapter 6)	Lunch out	Brownie Bites (Chapter 15)	Sweet and Sour Pork Skillet (Chapter 11) with Brown Rice and Vegetable Sauté (Chapter 13)
Day 6	Egg White Pancakes (Chapter 6)	Sweet and Sour Pork Skillet (Chapter 11) with Brown Rice and Vegetable Sauté (Chapter 13)	Brownie Bites (Chapter 15)	Dinner out
Day 7	Great Greek Omelet (Chapter 6)	Power Salad (Chapter 8)	One serving of fruit and 10 almonds	Crab Cakes with Sesame Crust (Chapter 12) and Honey Lemon Asparagus (Chapter 14)

A Basic Grocery List for Good Health

Starches:

- Corn tortillas
- High-fiber cereal (bran-based)
- Low-carb tortillas
- Oatmeal
- Rice cakes
- Shredded wheat, Cheerios
- Starchy vegetables and beans (corn, peas, pinto/black beans/chickpeas)
- Whole-wheat crackers
- Whole-wheat or multigrain bread and English muffins

Fruits (Fresh):

- Apples
- Avocados
- Bananas
- Berries
- Grapes
- Melons
- Oranges
- Pears

Vegetables (Fresh or Fresh-Frozen):

- Asparagus
- Basil
- Broccoli
- Carrots
- Cauliflower
- Celery
- Eggplant
- Green beans
- Mushrooms
- Spinach/lettuce
- Tomatoes
- Zucchini

Dairy:

- 2% cheese slices and shredded cheese
- 2% cottage cheese
- Fat-free half-and-half or soy/almond creamer (unsweetened)
- Fat-free or light cream cheese
- Greek yogurt
- Light spreadable cheese wedges
- Light string cheese
- Light yogurt
- Skim milk (light soy milk or unsweetened almond milk)

Meat/Poultry/Meat Substitutes:

- Canned tuna (packed in water)
- Chicken breasts
- Eggs or liquid egg whites
- Firm or extra-firm tofu
- Fish (fresh or frozen halibut, salmon, or tuna)
- Hummus
- Lean ground turkey
- Natural peanut butter or almond butter
- Turkey breast

Frozen Foods:

- Frozen chicken breast/fish fillets (unbreaded)
- Frozen edamame
- Frozen vegetables
- Low-sugar Popsicles
- Protein "hamburger"-style vegetable burgers

Beverages, Canned Foods, Condiments, Snack Foods:

- Dijon mustard
- Light air-popped popcorn
- Light mayonnaise
- Light whipped butter or margarine
- Lower-sugar jam
- Low-sodium chicken or vegetable broth
- Low-sodium soy sauce
- Nonstick cooking spray
- Nuts
- Olive oil
- Salsa
- Spices (cinnamon, garlic powder, onion powder, other dried spices without salt, pumpkin pie spice, vanilla extract)
- Tomato and marinara sauce
- Vinegar (rice, balsamic, red wine)

Online Pre-Diabetes and Diabetes Education Resources

American Council on Exercise (ACE)

A nonprofit organization that certifies fitness professionals and promotes safe and effective physical activity.

www.acefitness.org/fitfacts

American Diabetes Association

This site, maintained by the recognized authority on diabetes, is dedicated to providing up-to-date diabetes information, researching findings, and advocating for people with diabetes.

www.diabetes.org

Ask the Dietitian

Joanne Larsen, MS, RD, LD, maintains this site. You can use it to post specific diet-related questions or read the answers to questions from other visitors.

www.dietitian.com

CDC Division of Nutrition, Physical Activity, and Obesity

Research and resources for physical activity from the CDC.

www.cdc.gov/nccdphp/dnpao/state-local-programs/physicalactivity.html

DASH Eating Plan

Describes the DASH Eating Plan and its benefits, as well as tips and guidelines for following.

www.nhlbi.nih.gov/health-topics/dash-eating-plan

MyFitnessPal

A site (also available as an app) that enables you to track food and physical activity, and also includes an online community for social support.

www.myfitnesspal.com

National Diabetes Education Program (NDEP)

The NDEP helps translate the latest diabetes research into practical information for people with diabetes. Their website features many free, downloadable publications.

www.cdc.gov/diabetes/ndep/index.html

National Institute of Diabetes and Digestive and Kidney Diseases

A site for general diabetes information, where articles about many topics can be found.

www.niddk.nih.gov

National Institute on Aging

Exercise tips, plans, and resources for older adults.

www.nia.nih.gov

Oldways

A site that offers extensive information, resources, and recipes for the Mediterranean diet and other cultural eating patterns.

https://oldwayspt.org

SparkPeople

A free online site available for calorie and exercise tracking that has a strong online support network, as well as educational articles and videos.

www.sparkpeople.com

USDA ChooseMyPlate

A site developed by the United States Department of Agriculture (USDA) that discusses the MyPlate tool, which reviews and illustrates the five food groups and is the USDA's latest food guide symbol. It reviews all the food groups in detail, discusses portions and healthy choices, and there is also a section on physical activity. Recipes and other tools are available on the site as well.

www.choosemyplate.gov

US National Library of Medicine and National Institutes of Health/ Medline Plus

This site has research, references, interactive tutorials, consumer materials, and guidebooks to download or order online.

https://medlineplus.gov/diabetes.html

STANDARD **US/METRIC** MEASUREMENT CONVERSIONS

VOLUME CONVERSIONS

US Volume Measure	Metric Equivalent
⅛ teaspoon	0.5 milliliter
¼ teaspoon	1 milliliter
½ teaspoon	2 milliliters
1 teaspoon	5 milliliters
½ tablespoon	7 milliliters
1 tablespoon (3 teaspoons)	15 milliliters
2 tablespoons (1 fluid ounce)	30 milliliters
¼ cup (4 tablespoons)	60 milliliters
⅓ cup	90 milliliters
½ cup (4 fluid ounces)	125 milliliters
⅔ cup	160 milliliters
¾ cup (6 fluid ounces)	180 milliliters
1 cup (16 tablespoons)	250 milliliters
1 pint (2 cups)	500 milliliters
1 quart (4 cups)	1 liter (about)

WEIGHT CONVERSIONS

US Weight Measure	Metric Equivalent
½ ounce	15 grams
1 ounce	30 grams
2 ounces	60 grams
3 ounces	85 grams
¼ pound (4 ounces)	115 grams
½ pound (8 ounces)	225 grams
¾ pound (12 ounces)	340 grams
1 pound (16 ounces)	454 grams

OVEN TEMPERATURE CONVERSIONS

Degrees Fahrenheit	Degrees Celsius
200 degrees F	95 degrees C
250 degrees F	120 degrees C
275 degrees F	135 degrees C
300 degrees F	150 degrees C
325 degrees F	160 degrees C
350 degrees F	180 degrees C
375 degrees F	190 degrees C
400 degrees F	205 degrees C
425 degrees F	220 degrees C
450 degrees F	230 degrees C

BAKING PAN SIZES

American	Metric
8 × 1½ inch round baking pan	20 × 4 cm cake tin
9 × 1½ inch round baking pan	23 × 3.5 cm cake tin
11 × 7 × 1½ inch baking pan	28 × 18 × 4 cm baking tin
13 × 9 × 2 inch baking pan	30 × 20 × 5 cm baking tin
2 quart rectangular baking dish	30 × 20 × 3 cm baking tin
15 × 10 × 2 inch baking pan	30 × 25 × 2 cm baking tin (Swiss roll tin)
9 inch pie plate	22 × 4 or 23 × 4 cm pie plate
7 or 8 inch springform pan	18 or 20 cm springform or loose bottom cake tin
9 × 5 × 3 inch loaf pan	23 × 13 × 7 cm or 2 lb narrow loaf or pate tin
1½ quart casserole	1.5 liter casserole
2 quart casserole	2 liter casserole

Index

Note: Page numbers in **bold** indicate recipe category summaries.

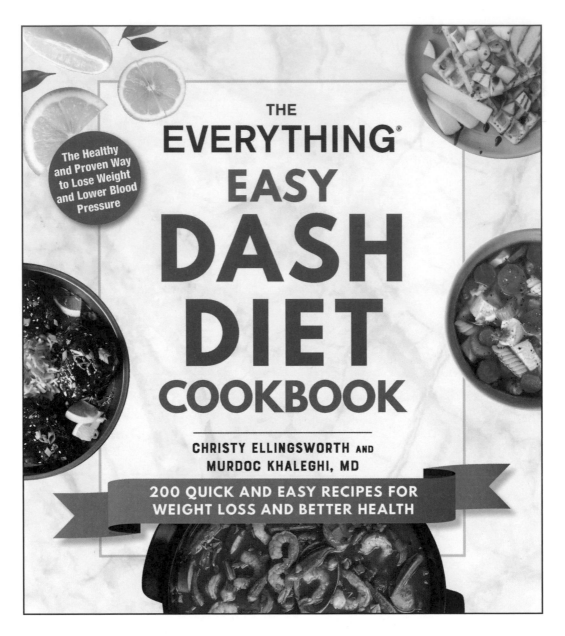
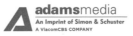